Medical Practice Management in the 21st Century

THE HANDBOOK

Marjorie A Satinsky MBA

with Randall T Curnow Jr MD MBA

Radcliffe Publishing

Oxford • New York

Radcliffe Publishing Ltd
18 Marcham Road
Abingdon
Oxon OX14 1AA
United Kingdom

www.radcliffe-oxford.com

Electronic catalogue and worldwide online ordering facility.

British Library Cataloguing in Publication Data

A catalogue record for this book is available from the British Library.
ISBN-10 1 84619 023 1
ISBN-13 978 1 84619 023 0

Typeset by Egan Reid Ltd, Auckland, New Zealand
Printed and bound by Alden (Malaysia)

Medical Practice Management in the 21st Century
THE HANDBOOK

This book is dedicated to
John A Fallon, MD, MBA, FACP

Table of Contents

Foreword   ix

Preface   x

About the Authors   xi

Acknowledgements   xii

Introduction   xiii

Section I: Getting Started

1 Creating a Strong Foundation for Your Practice   1

2 Organizing and Managing Your Practice   5

3 Business Planning   17

4 Marketing   27

Section II: Managing Finances

5 Introduction to Financial Management   39

6 Revenue Cycle Management   53

Section III: Recruiting and Managing Staff and Outside Resources

7 Human Resources   69

8 Physician Issues   89

9 Using Outsourcing Effectively   103

10 Hiring and Managing Consultants   113

Section IV: Improving Healthcare Delivery and Clinical Outcomes

11 Quality of Care   117

12 Using Information Technology to Enhance the Quality of Care, Operational
   Efficiency, and Revenue in Your Practice   129

Section V: Ensuring Compliance

13 Corporate Compliance   147

14 An Overview of HIPAA Compliance   159

15 HIPAA Privacy Rule and Security Rule Concepts   169

Appendix A: Steps for Creating a Strong Foundation   171

List of Additional Appendices Appearing only on the Website   185

Index   187

Foreword

In a world that is rapidly changing, physicians find that the business side of practicing medicine can lead to stress and anxiety. Running a successful and financially profitable practice is increasingly challenging. Many blame outside forces for the lack of success. "It is the government," "It is the insurer," "I cannot find good people." The blame game may lead to some emotional relief, but it does not solve the issues of surviving in a tough environment. Another common approach is presuming that working harder and seeing more patients will result in a better outcome. This leads to burn out and frustration. Working harder and longer doesn't address and correct. Behaving in the same old way produces the same old results.

A better method of addressing the challenges of managing a medical practice is to introduce sound business practices, including best practice, into your office. This approach requires that you are current and professional in the approach to the business of medicine. It involves the introduction of proven systems that involve all staff. Working as a team, you and your staff decide how to deal with the outside world of which you are a part. In my experience, most problems in the office are self-inflicted. It is likely that someone elsewhere has had a similar problem and found an effective way to solve it.

For clinicians, finding solutions to business problems is like learning to fly an airplane. If you are unfamiliar with practice management, the business of medicine can be a world of downdrafts, hard landings and bumpy rides. Before you learn to fly, you need a good flight manual. *Medical Practice Management in the 21st Century: the handbook* is such a manual. It is written by experienced people who have successfully dealt with practice management and taught it to practicing physicians. The authors take a pragmatic approach that will help streamline procedures, develop a digital office, and implement systems to ensure harmony among staff and patients. They know where the mountains are and how to avoid crashing into them.

This book is essential for any clinician planning to open a new practice or attempting to improve the quality and efficiency of an existing practice. Most practices run in routine crisis mode. If crisis is routine it is not crisis at all, but a failure of management to act. Using the pragmatic approach presented in this book will allow a clinician to get out of "routine crisis" and back to the profession of helping people. Utilizing this book will improve your health and the health of others. Read and learn . . .

John Bachman, MD
Sanders Professor of Primary Care
Mayo Clinic, Rochester
November 2006

Preface

As authors, we believe that mastering the art of medical practice management requires knowledge that most physicians don't learn in medical school, residency, or fellowship training. Successful practice management in the twenty-first century will require physicians to understand how to organize and manage a practice, manage their finances, recruit, work with, and manage people within and outside of the practice, improve healthcare delivery and clinical outcomes, and ensure compliance with federal, state, and local laws and regulations. Like clinical care, practice management also requires clinicians to understand how to enhance their knowledge on an ongoing basis.

Information on medical practice management is readily available on the Internet, in books and journal articles, and from professional associations. In our experiences as a consultant and physician who have managed our own practices and who help others do the same, inquisitive learners must painstakingly research one topic at a time. Most books and other learning tools have a single focus.

This book addresses multiple aspects of medical practice management. It offers both background information and practical tools. Our workbook format allows busy physicians to gain a basic understanding of many topics, determine strategies for their practices, and seek additional information when they want it. The supplementary material, including forms, worksheets, balance sheets, and contracts, can be found at www.radcliffe-oxford.com/medicalpracticemanagement.

The audience for the book is both physicians who need business guidance as they begin their careers and physicians who are already in practice and want to enhance their business skills. Many physicians can't afford, or choose not, to hire a professional practice administrator or manager; this book will help them assume managerial responsibilities with the same level of confidence that they bring to clinical care. Physicians in academic medical centers who manage departments, programs, or research studies can also benefit.

The goals of the book are to:

- guide physicians at various stages of their careers, in multiple specialties, and in different sized practices, in understanding the state-of-the-art of medical practice management

- identify the major topics with which physicians in management should be familiar

- for each of the major topics, provide helpful information and tools

- balance conceptual and practical information by using case studies, sample forms, and worksheets to illustrate important points

- provide suggested resources for those physicians who want to learn more.

Marjorie A Satinsky
Randall T Curnow, MD
November 2006

x

About the Authors

Marjorie A Satinsky, MBA is President of Satinsky Consulting, LLC, a consulting firm in Durham, NC. Prior to establishing her own company in 2002, she worked for 30 years in community and academic settings in both medical practices and hospitals. Working backwards chronologically, she ran a pediatric specialty practice in Chapel Hill, NC (Student Success Center of All Kinds of Minds, Inc.), served as President of a large Physician Hospital Organization (PHO) in Raleigh, NC, and was Duke Medical Center's Director of Managed Care Contracting and Operations. She held various hospital positions in Massachusetts and was the first hospital-based managed care director in that state. She also served on the Board and Executive Committee of the Tufts Associated Health Plan in Massachusetts and the Alice Aycock Poe Center for Health Education in North Carolina.

Ms Satinsky is the author of two books, *The Foundations of Integrated Care* (1998) and *An Executive Guide to Case Management Strategies* (1995), and numerous articles on medical practice management for the North Carolina Medical Board *Forum* and other professional journals. She is an Adjunct Faculty member at University of North Carolina School of Public Health. Ms Satinsky is a frequent speaker on topics related to medical practice management. She is a member of MGMA and a former Fellow of the American College of Healthcare Executives. Ms Satinsky has a BA from Brown University, an MA from University of Pennsylvania, and an MBA from the Wharton School, University of Pennsylvania.

Randall T Curnow, Jr, MD, MBA, CPE is President of Boylan Medical Associates in Raleigh, NC. He is a graduate of Oberlin College and University of Virginia School of Medicine. He did his residency training at Emory University School of Medicine and received his MBA from the University of Massachusetts, Amherst. As a member of the American College of Physician Executives, Dr Curnow was made Certified Physician Executive (CPE). He is also a member of the American College of Physicians, the American Medical Association, and the American College of Healthcare Executives. His book review, *Allies or Adversaries*, was published on the American College of Physician Executives web page.

Acknowledgements

Many people have assisted the authors with the development of this book. John A Fallon, MD of Blue Cross Blue Shield of Massachusetts, to whom this book is dedicated, has been a mentor and colleague for 20 years. When he took his first step in transitioning from clinical practice to medical practice management and integrated delivery systems, he searched for a way to feel as confident in the board room as he did in an exam room. He taught us the challenges that physicians in management encounter. Dale Breaden of the North Carolina Medical Board encouraged us to share our knowledge of medical practice management with North Carolina physicians and eventually with a wider audience.

Other healthcare professionals who contributed to this book are John W Bachman, MD; Sue Ellen Cox, MD; Morris Friedman, MD; Wilson Heyman; Damian McHugh, MD; Barnett Satinsky; Thomas Sena, MD; Carol Silverstein; Steven Shaber; Stephen Smith; Allen Wenner, MD; John Whelan, MD; and Randall Whitmeyer.

Special thanks go to Stan Wakefield for connecting us with Radcliffe Publishing, and to Gillian Nineham and Paula Jales, for their help in bringing this book to fruition. We also extend our deepest gratitude to Alice Saunders, who worked with us locally to organize a vast amount of information without losing our way.

Our families have provided ongoing support. Buzz, Fredda, Meagen, Sara, and Jonathan Satinsky, and Theresa, Ryan, and Colin Curnow have never wavered in their confidence and encouragement. We thank you all.

Introduction

Medical Practice Management in the 21st Century is divided into five sections: Getting Started, Managing Finances, Recruiting and Managing Staff and Outside Resources, Improving Healthcare Delivery and Clinical Outcomes, and Ensuring Compliance. We believe that a well run practice balances all five components, and so we recommend reading all five sections. Nonetheless, we have written each chapter as a separate entity, making it easy for you to focus on topics of particular interest. We have also put some of the tools and exhibits on a special website (www.radcliffe-oxford.com/medicalpracticemanagement) so you can customize the material for your practice.

Section I is *Getting Started*.

▶ Chapter 1 provides guidance in creating a *strong foundation* for your practice. It addresses the broad categories of activity that you should consider in managing a medical practice and identifies the necessary steps within each category. It guides your determination of responsibilities for different tasks and your placement of the tasks in a logical order.

▶ Chapter 2 is about *organization and management*. It helps you identify goals and priorities that you can translate into decisions about legal structure, affiliation, and relationships with physician colleagues. It also deals with practice structure and accountability.

▶ Chapter 3 is about *business planning*. It helps you develop a formal plan and use it appropriately. It suggests people who should participate in your business planning process. Finally, it identifies common challenges to successful business planning and ways in which you can overcome them.

▶ Chapter 4 is about *marketing*. It defines marketing and explains why you need it. It describes successful marketing and suggests individuals and groups toward which you should direct your efforts. It suggests techniques, including use of a practice website. It helps you measure the effectiveness of your marketing program, obtain help from external experts, and address legal and ethical constraints.

Section II is *Managing Finances*.

▶ Chapter 5 is an *introduction to financial management*. It explains the concept in layperson's language. It addresses concerns that often deter physicians from mastering the financial management of their practices. It suggests ways to learn more. It provides specific examples of information that you should review regularly. Finally, it provides steps you can take when you uncover problems in your practice.

▶ Chapter 6 is about *revenue cycle management*. It explains the term and suggests steps for developing a program. It suggests specific indicators and benchmarks that can help you manage revenue cycle management. It provides ways to maximize revenue from both patients and from managed care companies. It offers specific suggestions for protecting and enhancing your revenue. It provides guidance for dealing with your collection agency.

Finally, it explains how information technology can help you manage your revenue cycle management program and suggests resources for additional help.

Section III is *Recruiting and Managing Staff and Outside Resources*.

▶ Chapter 7 is about *human resources*. It outlines the federal, state, and local laws that affect your relationship with your employees. It addresses recruitment strategies, employee orientation, training, compensation, and design. It provides suggestions for encouraging job stability, addressing employee grievances, and developing a performance evaluation program. It provides guidance in handling disciplinary action, and resignations, terminations, and other departures from your practice. It offers suggestions for dealing with the diverse demographics in the twenty-first century workplace and suggests good resources on employee human resource management.

▶ Chapter 8 covers *physician issues*. It addresses physician recruitment, retention, orientation, compensation, performance evaluation, and departures from your practice. It offers guidance on learning more about physician issues.

▶ Chapter 9 is about *outsourcing*. It suggests functions that you can outsource to experienced external consultants and/or vendors, and it guides you in selecting those resources.

▶ Chapter 10 is about *hiring and managing consultants*. It suggests steps you can take ahead of time to find an individual and/or firm that meets your needs. It outlines the general characteristics of a good consultant and suggests steps for finding one. It discusses consultant charges and written agreements.

Section IV is *Improving Healthcare Delivery and Clinical Outcomes*.

▶ Chapter 11 is about *quality of care*. It explains quality and quality improvement. It describes the quality improvement programs that already exist. It suggests measurements that can help you compare your current status with post-improvement status. Finally, it suggests specific steps you can take within your own practice.

▶ Chapter 12 is about *using information technology* to enhance the quality of care, operational efficiency, and revenue in your practice. It describes four important information technology applications for your practice and the challenges in planning and implementing information technology to support your practice. It provides suggestions for internal work before you contact vendors and a step-by-step guide to reviewing your options and making decisions. It suggests keys to successful implementation of all information technology applications. Finally, it provides lessons learned from other practices and additional resources.

Section V is *Ensuring Compliance*.

▶ Chapter 13 is on *corporate compliance*. It explains the term and tells you why you need a compliance plan. It offers guidance in those aspects of your practice toward which to target your efforts. It describes the laws and regulations that affect corporate compliance and the penalties. It suggests steps to take to plan, implement, and maintain a corporate compliance program and identifies other laws and regulations with which your practice should comply.

▶ Chapter 14 is an overview of *compliance with the Health Insurance Portability and Accountability Act* of 1996 (HIPAA). It explains who must comply, the purpose and history of the act, the timetable for implementation, and ways in which the government enforces compliance with the HIPAA Privacy and HIPAA Security Rules. It describes the similarities and differences between Privacy and Security. It provides guidance in selecting your Privacy and Security Officials and suggests specific steps in a logical order that you should take to ensure compliance. Finally, it identifies factors that are likely to contribute to successful compliance and suggests additional resources on the Privacy and Security Rules.

▶ Chapter 15 explains the *HIPAA Privacy and Security Rule Concepts*. The terms in both rules may be new to you so you may want to use this chapter as a resource.

1 Creating a Strong Foundation for Your Practice

If you have ever built a house, you know that setting a firm foundation is essential. You don't want the walls or the roof to cave in when the first hurricane wind blows your way. The same principle applies to your medical practice. If you set the foundation properly, you can position yourself to build a strong practice. The healthcare environment is always in a state of flux, and you want to be ready for whatever comes your way.

Likewise, if you are already actively involved or are assuming additional managerial responsibilities in an existing medical practice, you should regularly monitor your structural foundation. No practice can survive or thrive if it stands on shaky ground.

Here are four questions about medical practice management that are important in all situations:

⦁ What broad categories of activities should you perform in order to manage a medical practice?

⦁ Within each broad category of activities, what specific steps should you take?

⦁ Who should be responsible for accomplishing each task?

⦁ If you are opening a new practice or are moving to a new location, what tasks should you complete before you open or move your practice, and what tasks can wait until after you start to see patients?

Broad categories of activities

An ideal medical practice balances organization and management, financial management, recruiting and managing staff and outside resources, improving healthcare delivery and clinical outcomes, and ensuring compliance. To start and sustain a balanced practice, focus your efforts on these five categories and spread your efforts among them.

⦁ *Organization and Management (OM):* It goes without saying that you must decide exactly what services you want to provide to patients both when you open a practice and as you continue to grow. As a primary care physician or specialist, you have choices. You can provide basic services such as office visits and surgery, and/or you can offer your patients the convenience of getting laboratory tests, radiological exams, therapies, and other services on your premises. You may want to start simply and then add services as your financial viability grows. You don't need to do everything right away.

How will you set up your practice or change your existing practice structure? You can incorporate or not, and your attorney can give you good advice on which method is most suitable for you. When you decide on your structure, you'll want to make sure that you have the appropriate supporting legal documents.

If you are in solo practice or planning to work with one or more colleagues, give some thought to physician issues. Will you have partners and/or employees? How will you compensate yourself and the other physicians in your practice? If your arrangements with other physicians don't work out as you planned, how will you terminate these relationships?

What administrative structure is most appropriate for your practice? Do you and your physician colleagues want to play an active managerial role or are you comfortable delegating a portion of this work to a professional practice administrator or manager? If physicians do have managerial responsibilities, how will you decide who does what, and will you pay physicians for the time they devote to administration?

Your practice is a business. Have you developed a strategic business plan, a supporting budget, and an implementation plan that specifies your mission, values, goals, strategies, and action steps? If you do strategic business planning when you set your practice up and thereafter on a regular basis, you can create a clear road map for everyone to follow.

Do you know the importance of marketing your practice? The messages you communicate within your practice to your patients, physicians, and staff, and your external communications with medical colleagues, healthcare organizations, your community, and potential patients are important, not just fluff. A well-designed website with functional capabilities can be an important tool.

▶ *Financial Management (FM):* From the very start your goal will be to generate as much revenue as you can, keep careful control of expenses, and do financial planning for your practice and yourself. You'll generate revenue from multiple sources that include but are not limited to public and private payers, ancillary services, and/or real estate. You'll have capital and operating expenses. Working with your Certified Public Accountant (CPA), you'll want to support the strategic portion of your business plan with operating and capital budgets, a balance sheet, and cash flow statements. You'll want to put in place good revenue cycle management practices that include contract negotiation with third party payers, patient registration, coding, and billing and collections.

▶ *Managing Staff and Outside Resources (HR):* Your success depends on both your own knowledge and experience in caring for patients and on your clinical and administrative team. A major decision will be whether or not to hire a professional practice administrator or manager. You'll want to hire, train, reward, and retain individuals who help you deliver the best possible medical care and service to your patients and colleagues and who work well as a team. You'll need good job descriptions, a compensation package that you can afford, and a performance evaluation system. For your own protection, you'll need a comprehensive Employee Handbook and a standard orientation package. With respect to physicians, you'll need systems for recruitment, employment, adding partners, compensation, and departures from your practice.

▶ *Improving Healthcare Delivery and Clinical Outcomes (DO):* You may like to think your patients judge you solely on the quality of care that you provide, but in truth, they scrutinize your processes for delivering care and your workflow as carefully as they assess the clinical services that they receive. They also notice the information technology that supports your practice – i.e., your practice management system, your website, electronic health records (EHR), e-prescribing, and the integration among all these applications.

‣ As your practice grows, you'll want to make sure that both care of individual patients and of groups of patients meets appropriate and evidence-based standards and that you can document what you have done. Professional organizations already require demonstrated competency in quality and quality improvement. The federal government is now funding demonstration programs relating to quality of care and encouraging physicians throughout the country to voluntarily report quality information. The handwriting is on the wall, and, within the foreseeable future, public and private payers will relate financial incentives to quality. Every physician believes that he/she provides excellent care – but can you prove it? Make sure you understand both quality care and quality improvement and that you put in place systems that will help you track information about your patients. Use that information to enhance the good care that you already provide and document what you do.

‣ *Compliance (C):* Compliance with federal, state, and local regulations isn't optional; it's an essential component of risk management. You need to understand the statutes that govern Medicare and Medicaid fraud and abuse, anti-kickback, anti-discrimination, and HIPAA. More important, you need to be proactive in your compliance activities.

A step-by-step guide to setting up or improving your practice

Now that you know the broad categories of practice management, you are ready to take specific steps. If you want to create and/or maintain a balanced practice, it is advisable to mix the steps from the different categories, rather than concentrating on one category at a time. If you concentrate on one category at a time, you may find yourself unable to move ahead because you have placed the proverbial cart before the horse.

The list in Appendix A describes each step that you need to take at three different points in time – when you start a practice, if and when you move, and when you want to assess your current practice and make improvements. The list provides guidance for internal and/or external responsibility. Sometimes you and/or your practice administrator/manager can do the work, but in other situations, you may want to seek assistance from one or more consultants external to your practice. If you are starting a new practice or moving to a new location, you should complete most of the tasks on the list before you open your doors or move. In some cases, you can wait until after you have seen your first patient. The code beside each task identifies the category into which the task fits: Organization and Management (OM); Financial Management (FM); Managing Staff and Outside Resources (HR); Improving Healthcare Delivery and Clinical Outcomes (DO); and Compliance (C).

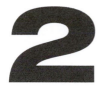 # Organizing and Managing Your Practice

Many books on practice management bury chapters on practice organization and management at the end of the book as if these topics were footnotes to more important subjects. If you stop to think about it, however, the way in which you organize and manage your practice impacts everything that you do, so why not consider it sooner rather than later? If you make thoughtful decisions about practice organization before problems arise, you will be in a much better position to address both anticipated and unanticipated situations.

Your decisions on practice organization should address at least the following five topics:

- What's important to you: The practice setting that you choose should reflect your preferences for collegiality, willingness to take risk, and interest in managing a small business.

- Legal decisions: What type of practice and legal entity are best for you, and what documents do you need to support your decisions?

- Affiliation decisions: Will your practice affiliate with organizations in your community that collaborate with and/or provide support to physician practices? If so, what documents do you need to support your decisions?

- Physician decisions: If your practice has more than one physician, how will you relate to each other? Will you be partners, or will some of you be employees? As you grow and recruit additional physicians, will you bring them in as partners and/or employees?

- Structure and accountability: Given the scope of practice management, how will you manage your practice? What roles will you, other physicians, and your practice administrator/manager play? Will you outsource some of your responsibilities to outside consultants?

What's important to you?

You've had opportunities during your medical school, residency, fellowship training, and actual practice to work in different private practice settings. Whether you are just starting out in your medical career or contemplating a change, it's essential to think about your own needs. Here are questions you should ask yourself before you make decisions about practice organization.

- Will I be comfortable practicing as a solo physician or will I prefer an environment where I work closely with colleagues in my specialty or in multiple specialties?

- Am I willing to take the financial risk that accompanies starting a practice?

▶ Am I willing to assume an active role in managing a small business, or do I prefer that someone else assumes the responsibility for management?

▶ Am I willing to share practice management responsibilities with other physicians and/or a practice administrator/manager?

Keep your answers to these questions in mind as you address your decisions regarding type of practice, legal entity, affiliations with other organizations, and management.

Legal decisions

When you set up your practice and/or make a change later in your career, you will have choices about your type of practice, about the legal entity that you create, and about the type(s) of physician support and other organizations with which you affiliate. The choices are described below. Legal counsel can give you more specific information and advice.

Type of practice

You can set yourself up as a solo practitioner, a single specialty group, or a multi-specialty group:[1,2]

▶ *Solo Practice:* Physicians who have completed their training and who have an entrepreneurial spirit may choose solo practice as an entry into the field of medical practice. Solo practice is a way to test the waters of medical practice, particularly if you are new in a community and have not worked with other physicians who practice there. Even if solo practice is not your choice when you first go into practice, you may select this option after you have had the experience of working with colleagues. Regardless of when you make the solo practice decision, keep in mind that you will have full responsibility for the ownership and operations of your practice. You will probably want to make coverage arrangements with colleagues in other practices. With respect to employees, a supportive team that is comfortable with multi-tasking and an experienced practice management consultant are essential.

▶ *Single Specialty Group:* You may prefer to work with colleagues who practice in your specialty rather than as a solo physician. Three advantages of a single specialty group over solo practice are the opportunity to share call coverage, the potential leverage in managed care contracting, and economies of scale in operations. The single specialty option can be attractive to a new physician who wants to learn the ropes of the business of medicine. The famous medical school adage, "See one, do one, teach one," applies to management as well as to clinical care.

▶ *Multi-specialty Group:* Some physicians prefer a multi-specialty group to a single specialty group so they can refer patients to colleagues within their own organization. The advantages over solo practice are related to call coverage, managed care contracting, and operational economies of scale. A physician who joins a well-established multi-specialty group will have no start-up costs and will have the advantages of a generous benefit package and time off for vacation and continuing education. One disadvantage of the multi-specialty group model can be the distribution of revenue among various specialty groups. Revenue distribution is always complicated, and this model presents the greatest challenge.

Legal entity

You have choices about the legal entity you create for your medical practice. Each option has advantages and disadvantages. Pay particular attention to differences in taxation, protection against liability judgments, dissolution requirements, degree of autonomy, and business risk. There is no right answer; you need to select the model that best meets your needs. In some situations, medical group practices establish more than one legal entity to manage different aspects of their business.

Medical practices fall into two broad categories, unincorporated and incorporated.[3] Most but not all physicians choose incorporation. Unincorporated set-ups include sole proprietorships, general partnerships, limited partnerships, and limited liability partnerships. Incorporated set-ups are more formal and costly than unincorporated practices and also offer more benefits. Their main advantage is protection from personal liability for professional acts of colleagues.

▶ *Sole Proprietorship:* Sole proprietorship is the easiest and least expensive way to start a practice. A single individual owns and operates the practice either in his/her own name or in a name chosen. The physician-owner can employ physician and non-physician staff and/or arrange for staffing through a management services organization (MSO). He/she can also avoid taxation requirements by contracting with other physicians as independent contractors. The physician-owner signs all contracts and collects all revenues in his/her name. He/she is liable for all obligations of the practice, and personal assets can be claimed to settle a lawsuit against the business. Unlike other forms of practice organization, sole proprietorships are not formally regulated. Nonetheless, state law may require that you register the name of the business. With respect to taxation, the physician owner reports practice revenues as personal income. If you start with a sole proprietorship and decide to change your structure, conversion to an S corporation or a C corporation and sometimes to a limited liability partnership or limited liability company does not trigger taxes.

▶ *General Partnership:* A partnership is an association of two or more people who act as co-owners of a for-profit business. With respect to medical practices, the number of partners is unlimited. The partners can employ and/or contract with other physicians. State law regulates general partnerships. The partners share equally in the profits and losses of the business, or, by agreement, they can make other arrangements based on the revenues and expenses generated by each of the partners. Because each partner assumes joint and several liability for the obligations of the partnership, he/she can incur obligations for which all partners are liable.

Although there are ways to limit the risk, some physicians choose another option rather than entering into a general partnership. The grounds for dissolution should be spelled out in the partnership agreement. Often, when a general partnership dissolves upon a triggering event such as the death or retirement of a partner, the remaining partners decide to continue the practice by forming a new partnership.

It is easier to establish a general partnership than a corporation. There's no requirement for a corporate charter or other statutory requirements. There are no fees for filing or for forming and operating the partnership. With respect to taxation, provided that a partnership lacks two of four corporate characteristics, the profits and losses of a partnership are attributed to the individual partners, so there is no double taxation as there is with corporations.

▶ *Limited Partnership:* A limited partnership is similar to a general partnership, with an important difference. The liability of each limited partner is limited to that partner's capital contribution so long as the limited partner doesn't participate in daily management. Each state has its own requirements for establishing a limited partnership. As with a general partnership, the income of the partnership is taxed to each partner. There is no double taxation so long as the partnership lacks two of four corporate characteristics. If a trigger event such as death, retirement, or resignation dissolves the limited partnership, the partnership can be reformed.

▶ *Limited Liability Partnership:* Some but not all states authorize the creation of LLPs, general partnerships that have been modified to eliminate each partner's personal liability for the debts and obligations of the partners arising from the errors, omissions, negligence, incompetence, or malfeasance committed in the course of the partnership business by another partner or partnership representatives. A partner's business investment, however, is not protected if someone successfully sues the practice and the award exceeds insurance limits.[3] State law governs the establishment of LLPs, and most states require annual renewal of LLP status. An LLP is not subject to double taxation so long as the partnership lacks two of four corporate characteristics. Make sure not to confuse a limited liability partnership with a limited partnership established to invest in real estate or equipment leasing; they are not the same.[3]

▶ *Limited Liability Company:* An LLC is an unincorporated organization where the owners' liability is limited to their investment in the organization. The owners are treated as partners for taxation purposes. Most states have legislation regulating the formation and regulation of LLCs, and some states do not allow physicians to form LLCs. With respect to taxation, most LLCs are taxed as partnerships. A triggering event such as a death or resignation generally requires dissolution of the LLC, but the Internal Revenue Service (IRS) allows a majority of the remaining members to decide to continue.

▶ *Corporation:* A corporation is a public or private artificial person or legal entity with an identity distinct from that of its owners. A corporation can be public or private. If it is private, it is characterized by: limited liability, continuity of existence, transferability of ownership, and centralized management. Although there are exceptions to the limited liability of investors, investors are not personally liable for corporate obligations. Nonetheless, investors' initial obligations can be used to satisfy corporate financial obligations. Corporate officers and directors have two important fiduciary duties, the duty of care in managing corporate affairs and the duty of loyalty requiring directors and officers to act in the interest of the corporation rather than in their own interests. Directors and officers must also refrain from profiting from business opportunities that belong to the corporation. With respect to dissolution, with a corporation, ownership interest is transferable, thus allowing continuity of existence.

▶ *Professional Corporation:* A PC (or Professional Association/PA in some states) is similar to a general corporation with some differences. It is important to check state law. Unlike general corporations, PCs do not have free transferability of ownership interests, and in most cases, transferability of ownership is restricted to licensed professionals. Physician stockholders in a PC have limited liability for the ordinary business obligations of the group practice and are liable only for the amount of their investment in the PC. Nonetheless, physicians remain personally liable for medical malpractice and other torts arising from the practice of medicine. States vary in their requirements for the formation and regulation of PCs. Corporations have a tax disadvantage in that there is double taxation. The corporation is taxed on corporate income and the individual shareholder is taxed a second time on dividends and other distributions. Shareholders are not taxed on undistributed corporate profits. Good accounting advice can suggest ways to avoid the double taxation dilemma.

An alternative for the PC/PA is to qualify as a subchapter S corporation which is then taxed as a partnership. With this alternative, each shareholder is charged with a proportionate share of the profits/losses, and that amount is reported on the individual shareholder's personal income tax. There's no double taxation. An S corporation also makes it easier for a physician to sell his/her share of the practice.[3] A minor disadvantage of an S corporation is that, with the exception of health insurance, there is no tax write-off for benefits.

Affiliation decisions

Depending on the community in which your practice is located, you may have opportunities to establish one or more relationships between your practice and organizations that collaborate with and/or provide support to medical practices. Common examples are Group Practices without Walls, Independent Practice Associations (IPAs), Management Services Organizations (MSOs), Physician Hospital Organizations (PHOs), networks, and integrated delivery systems.

▶ *Group Practices without Walls:* Physicians keep their separate practice locations but become employees of a new corporation. Administrative services are managed or contracted centrally. Although the goal of this type of affiliation is to reduce overhead, the strategy does not always succeed because physicians retain their existing overhead structures. A well-known example of a failed group practice without walls is the Sacramento Sierra Medical Group in California, which at one time had more than 70 locations.[4]

▶ *Independent Practice Associations (IPAs):* Independent Practice Associations are legal entities of physicians and physician groups. The purpose is negotiation of contracts with those managed care companies that are willing to deal with physician organizations. Member physicians maintain their own practices and generally perform their own administrative services.

▶ *Management Service Organizations (MSOs):* A Management Services Organization provides administrative and management services to physicians on a contractual basis. Services that MSOs typically provide are practice management, marketing, managed care contracting, planning and implementation of management information systems, purchasing, facilities management, accounting, billing, and human resources.

▶ *Physician Hospital Organizations (PHOs):* In a PHO arrangement, physicians and hospitals collaborate for the purposes of managed care contracting, quality improvement, and information technology. The physicians in the organization may also be organized into an IPA or other physician arrangement. Alternatively, individual practices may be part of the PHO. There's no standard form for a PHO, and PHOs may be for-profit, a partnership, or another type of organization.

▶ *Networks:* In some communities, physicians in different organizational models link together in a network form in order to leverage their numbers in managed care contracting. Networks may collaborate with hospital systems to form an integrated delivery system.

▶ *Integrated Delivery Systems:* Integrated healthcare systems are organized delivery (and sometimes financing) that provides comprehensive health services to a defined population. In an integrated system, the different parts of the system work together to achieve economies of scale and other synergies to a degree not achieved by other delivery mechanisms. The term is often misused to describe any system that combines some aspects of delivery and financing.[5]

Regardless of your choices of structure for your group and affiliations with other organizations, make sure you have in place the appropriate supporting documents. Just like marriages, most practice start-ups and relationships with other healthcare organizations begin in an environment of good feeling. There's no way to predict what will happen over time within your own practice, within your community, or at state and national levels. It is essential to protect yourself and the others with whom you deal. Create a worksheet like the sample in Exhibit 2.1 so you can list the documents required for your particular situation. Your attorney can provide guidance.

EXHIBIT 2.1 Sample worksheet for identifying documents needed for legal entities and affiliations[4,1]

LEGAL ENTITY/AFFILIATION	REQUIRED DOCUMENTS
Sole Proprietorship	
General Partnership	
Limited Partnership	
Limited Liability Partnership	
Limited Liability Company	
Corporation	
Professional Corporation/Association	
Group Practice without Walls	
Independent Practice Association	
Management Service Organization	
Physician Hospital Organization (PHO)	
Network	
Integrated Delivery System	

Decisions about relationships with other physicians in your practice

Regardless of the type of practice and legal entity that you have selected and decisions that you make about affiliations between your practice and other organizations in your community, you will need to address the relationships between or among the physicians within your own practice. Are you creating a partnership? How many partners do you want? As you grow, will you employ physicians during a trial period before making partnership available to them?

Will one or more of the physician partners have management responsibilities? If so, what skills will you want that individual to have and how will you compensate him/her for time spent on administrative duties? Exhibit 2.2 describes the approach that Cornwallis Internal Medicine chose and the resulting problems.

EXHIBIT 2.2 Challenges at Cornwallis Internal Medicine

Cornwallis Internal Medicine is a multi-specialty group practice located in Southern Heaven, a southern town with a major university. The practice has existed for more than 25 years. Currently, four of its eight physicians specialize in gastroenterology and the others practice general internal medicine. The founding partners have all retired, and none of the current partners wants to assume long-term responsibility for running the practice. The physicians have agreed on a quarterly rotation for the important position of Managing Partner. Other partners share some of the administrative responsibilities. The practice manager has historically concentrated on daily operations and has not assumed a leadership role in guiding the practice. On paper, the partners appear to be managing their practice, but in reality, they are collaborating in avoiding responsibility. Accounts receivable are out of control. Managed care contracts have not been renegotiated in several years, and the practice has purchased an expensive Electronic Medical Record system under the false impression that the federal government required the purchase. The physicians are now struggling with EHR implementation. Cornwallis Internal Medicine's governance and management structures are barriers to the efficient operation of the practice.

Here are some suggestions for dealing with other physicians in your practice:

- If you have one or more physician partners, make sure your attorney draws up a partnership agreement for you at the very outset. Make sure all the partners are clear about expectations.

- If you expect to grow by adding physicians to your practice, consider starting new physicians as salaried employees. Give your new physicians the opportunity to work in the practice and in your community before you make a commitment to partnership. Make sure this trial period is clear up front, and develop specific criteria that you will use to evaluate readiness for partnership. Examples are: professional competence, group relations and participation, financial performance, and other characteristics such as communication skills and commitment to the practice.[4]

- If one or more physicians will act as the Managing Partner, develop specific criteria for selection. Here is a good starting point: professional credibility with peers, personal integrity, effective communications skills (listening, speaking, and writing), ability to think in terms of process and systems, leadership skills (envisioning the future, guiding the skill development of others, framing and facilitating conversations), commitment to team building, skill in negotiations and conflict resolution, interest in quality management, understanding of finance and managed care, and willingness to pursue advanced management training as needed.[6,7]

Decisions about practice structure and accountability

One of the most important decisions that you'll make about your practice is about the management. Who's in charge, and what does he/she manage? What role will the partners play? Will you hire a practice administrator or practice manager, and if so, what will be his/her responsibilities? Will you manage everything from within your practice, or will you outsource one or more functions to an external expert or consultant?

When you consider your options for practice management, you may be tempted to start with people rather than with a good understanding of the scope of medical practice management. If you start by looking at major topics and tasks, you will gain a better overview of everything that you need to do and make better choices about the division of responsibilities.

If you're not clear on the scope of medical practice management, review the framework that is used by MGMA (Medical Group Management Association), the professional organization for group practice managers (www.mgma.com). MGMA lists eight areas of proficiency for medical practice managers. Assume responsibility yourself and/or delegate the tasks within each of these areas. The eight areas are:

1　Financial management
2　Human resource management
3　Planning and marketing
4　Information technology
5　Risk management
6　Governance and organizational dynamics
7　Business and clinical operations
8　Professional responsibility.

As you determine how to divide responsibility for the various aspects of your practice, remember that there is no ideal way to make this decision. The right decision is what works in your unique situation, given your needs and the capabilities of your physicians and staff. For each area of proficiency, decide which person/persons can best understand the subject matter, think strategically and critically, and learn new information on an ongoing basis. Don't presume that a single individual must handle each and every task. Dividing responsibilities is fine, provided you know who is responsible for each task.

Here are questions for each area of proficiency that you should address when you set up your practice or, if you are already in practice, when you review the management and organization that you have in place. Be proactive. Don't be like so many practices that ignore questions about structure and responsibility until they encounter serious problems. By then it is too late, and they have to simultaneously tackle the structure of the practice, the suitability of individual staff members for particular jobs, and the problems themselves.

Financial management questions

▶ Who is responsible for revenue cycle management, including patient registration, coding, billing, and collections?

▶ Who ensures that your practice is coding in compliance with federal and state regulations?

▶ Who pays the bills?

▶ Who has check-signing authority?

▶ Who manages your accounts receivable?

▶ Who determines and enforces your collections policy?

▶ Who reviews end-of-month financial information provided by your accountant and by your practice management system in order to analyze it, identify problems, and recommend corrective action?

▶ Who establishes financial performance goals for your practice?

▶ Who benchmarks your financial performance against industry standards for your specialty?

▶ Who creates the capital and operating budgets for your practice?

▶ Who negotiates your managed care contracts and handles any problems that occur with the various payers?

Human resource management questions

▶ Who is in charge of physician recruitment, including but not limited to recruitment, interviewing, reference checks, completion of appropriate legal documents, credentialing, and mentoring?

▶ Who develops job descriptions for clinical and administrative staff?

▶ Who sets your salary scales for clinical and administrative staff?

▶ Who recruits and hires administrative and clinical staff?

▶ Who creates and maintains a Personnel Handbook containing policies and procedures for your practice?

▶ Who determines and documents the benefit package that you offer to partners and employees?

▶ Who creates and implements a performance evaluation system for your practice?

▶ Who creates a clear policy for terminating employees?

▶ Who determines if and when you seek external legal guidance regarding human resource issues?

Planning and marketing questions

▶ Who develops and updates your practice's strategic business plan?

▶ Who develops and implements an annual operating plan that is consistent with your business plan?

▶ Who ensures that the goals and objectives for individual members of your practice are consistent with your business and operating plans?

▶ Who makes sure that you infuse a patient focus into the operations of your practice so that marketing becomes everyone's responsibility?

▶ Who creates and implements your satisfaction surveys for patients and medical colleagues and ensures that you act on the results?

▶ Who creates and maintains a practice website as a means of communicating with your patients and medical colleagues?

▶ Who develops and maintains a patient information package that you distribute to all patients?

▶ Who develops brochures, newsletters, and other printed material for your practice?

▶ Who determines how you will relate to physicians, hospitals, and other healthcare organizations in your community?

▶ Who makes decisions about your participation in community activities, such as the Chamber of Commerce, the boards of non-profit organizations, health fairs, etc.?

Information technology questions

▶ Who is responsible for developing an information technology management strategy that includes but is not limited to your practice management system, your website, electronic health records, e-prescribing, your telephone system, and the relationships among these systems?

▶ Who maintains your hardware and software?

▶ Who are your HIPAA Privacy and Security Officials, and how does this person(s) make sure that you comply with the appropriate rules?

▶ If you are using an external information technology consultant, who in your practice provides guidance and feedback?

Risk management questions

▶ Who is your compliance officer?

▶ Who creates and maintains your Compliance Plan?

▶ Who monitors compliance?

Governance and organizational dynamics questions

▶ How are the partners involved in the management of your practice? Do you have a Managing Partner and/or do the partners share responsibility for management?

▶ If you have a practice administrator/manager, what are his/her responsibilities?

▶ Do you have clear guidelines for the way in which the practice administrator/manager relates to the partners in managing the practice?

▶ Do you have regular meetings of the partners and the Executive Committee?

▶ Do you have regular staff meetings?

▶ Who decides if and when you will use outside consultants?

▶ When you use outside consultants, what is the accountability?

▶ Do you have clear lines of authority and supervision in your practice?

Business and clinical operations questions

▶ Who determines the work flow process?

▶ If there are problems in work flow, who in your practice assumes responsibility for understanding the issues and taking corrective action?

▶ Who in your practice makes sure that the business and clinical operations support each other?

▶ Who is responsible for the flow of information in your practice?

▶ Who makes sure that you use available clinical and financial information to continuously improve your practice?

Professional responsibility questions

▶ Who sets professional standards for the clinical and administrative members of your practice?

▶ Who sets expectations for professional growth and development for everyone in your practice?

▶ How do you monitor compliance with professional standards for your partners and for your clinical and administrative staff?

▶ When your practice is confronted with a problem that it has not previously encountered, how do you go about finding a solution?

As you review these questions, document the decisions that you make about responsibilities. Below is a shortened version of Exhibit 2.3, which contains a sample responsibility list that can serve as a convenient reference when questions about accountability arise within your practice. The entire exhibit can be found on the website link www.radcliffe-oxford.com/medicalpracticemanagement.

EXHIBIT 2.3 Sample list of management responsibilities in a medical practice

TASK	PHYSICIAN	PRACTICE ADMIN/ MGR	PHYSICIAN AND PR.ADMN/MGR
FINANCIAL MANAGEMENT			
Revenue cycle management			
Coding compliance			
HUMAN RESOURCES MANAGEMENT			
Physician recruitment, interviewing, reference checks, legal documents, credentialing, mentoring			
Development/maintenance of job descriptions			
PLANNING AND MARKETING			
Development and updating of strategic business plan			
Development and implementation of annual operating plan			
INFORMATION TECHNOLOGY			
Development of information technology strategy			
Maintenance of hardware and software			

(*continued*)

TASK	PHYSICIAN	PRACTICE ADMIN/ MGR	PHYSICIAN AND PR.ADMN/MGR
COMPLIANCE			
Designation of compliance officer			
Development and maintenance of compliance plan			
MANAGEMENT AND GOVERNANCE			
Designation of Managing Partner(s)			
Determination of responsibilities of practice administrator/ manager			
CLINICAL OPERATIONS			
Determination and ongoing analysis of work flow process			
Determination and ongoing analysis of information flow			
PROFESSIONAL RESPONSIBILITY			
Setting professional standards for clinical and administrative members of workforce			
Monitoring compliance with professional standards			

References

1 Eldridge J (VP and Publisher), Conner C (Editorial Director, Health Law). *Medical Group Practice, Legal and Administrative Guide*. New York: Aspen Publishers; 1999–2003.
2 Paulus KH. Organizational Options Available to Physicians. In: Silver JK. *The Business of Medicine*. Philadelphia: Hanley & Belfus, Inc; 1998.
3 Murray D. S corp, C corp, LLC, LLP – which is best? *Medical Economics*. March 5, 2004: 81: 44.
4 Benedict G. *The Development and Management of Medical Groups*. Englewood, CO: MGMA; 1996.
5 Satinsky MA. *The Foundations of Integrated Care. Facing the Challenges of Change*. Chicago: American Hospital Publishing, Inc; 1998.
6 Pollard J. *The Physician Manager in Group Practice*. Englewood, CO: MGMA; 1995.
7 Alberts M. Business and Management Training for Physicians. In: Silver JK. *The Business of Medicine*. Philadelphia: Hanley & Belfus, Inc; 1998.

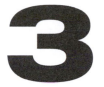 # Business planning

Think what havoc you would create for your family if you started out on a vacation with no idea of your destination or route. Apply that same principle to your medical practice and the stakes are higher. You jeopardize the likelihood that your practice will grow and thrive.

This chapter will answer the following questions:

▶ What is a business plan and why should you have one?

▶ What information should your business plan contain?

▶ How can you use your plan after you complete it?

▶ Who should participate in the planning process?

▶ When should you develop your business plan?

▶ What steps should you take and in what order?

▶ What are keys to a successful business planning process?

▶ What are common challenges to successful business planning and how can you overcome them?

What is a business plan and why should you have one?

Your business plan shows you the current status of your practice, where you are heading, and how financial and human capital will enable it to meet its goals. It helps you, your partners, and your staff to understand the relationships between the external environment and your unique medical practice. The information that is contained in your business plan is only part of its value. The process of developing the plan is important too. Your practice and external consultants create the plan so you can reach consensus on the direction in which your practice is going, the financing for that direction, the specific steps you will need to take, and on accountability and responsibility.

Sad to say, most physicians roll their eyes at the concept of a medical practice as a business. "I am a physician, not a businessman [or businesswoman]," is a common response to the suggestion of business planning. "I became a physician so I could avoid stuff like this," is another reaction. Yet a business plan should not be a foreign concept to physicians since it closely resembles components of the scientific method. A business plan forces management to create a hypothesis for a business strategy, to evaluate the underlying assumptions, and determine the fiscal, market, and non-market steps that are needed to make the strategy successful.

You need a business plan because people are human. You may think everyone in your practice agrees on goals and values, priorities, action steps, financial support, and delegation of responsibilities. In most cases, there is no consensus. You need a plan to keep everyone moving in harmony toward goals that you agree are appropriate for your practice.

What information should your business plan contain?

A good business plan has three essential components: a *strategic plan* that lays out broad direction, a *financial plan* that supports your strategic plan, and an *implementation plan* that specifies priorities and accountabilities. For simplicity's sake, this chapter will talk about all three components as if they were a single business plan.

The strategic component of your plan should have five sections: mission, vision, values, goals, and strategies. Your *mission* is your purpose for existing. Why are you in practice? What services do you want to provide to your patients? The answer may not always be clear. For example, the partners in a surgical practice may have different opinions about the percentage of effort devoted to general surgery versus specialty areas. If you don't articulate and work through your differences during your planning process, individual physicians in your practice may make decisions that have a negative impact on your patient care. What if one physician wants to concentrate on breast surgery and refuses to cover for patients of partners who specialize in other areas? The issue is less about coverage than about failure to agree on practice mission.

Your *vision* is your dream for tomorrow. Where do you want to be three to five years from now? Do you want to shift the emphasis of the services that you provide for patients so that you become more specialized? Do you want to provide additional services? Do you want to remain in your current location? Do you want to open satellite offices? Do you want to collaborate with other physicians and healthcare organizations in ways that are different from what you are currently doing? How do you want information technology to support the growth of your practice? Defining your vision will answer these questions and others.

Your *values* are your beliefs both as an organization and as individuals. What is your focus? Are you committed to staying on focus, or are you willing to deviate if new and interesting opportunities arise? What patient needs do you want to meet? Will you be active participants in community clinics that provide healthcare to patients who don't qualify for government assistance but can't afford to pay for care? What is your approach to collaboration with other physicians and healthcare organizations in your community? What is your style of financial management; are you risk-takers, risk averse, or somewhere in between the two extremes? What is your attitude toward your staff? Are you committed to personal growth and development, or are you more interested in hiring the least expensive employees that you can recruit? Are you committed to excellence in everything that you do? What is your approach toward innovation? How do you differentiate yourself from your competitors?

Identify major *goal categories* and then list specific goals in each category. Your goal categories might be practice organization and management, quality and quality improvement, financial management, human resources, practice operations, and compliance. Once you list the goals in each category, specify time frames. What do you want to accomplish this coming year, within three years, and within five years? Then list the *projects* related to each goal. Move on to *barriers and opportunities*, and finally to *strategies*.

Your *strategies* are your approaches for addressing the barriers and opportunities that you have identified. For example, if your goal is to introduce a practice website and electronic health records into your practice, you surely have opportunities. If some of your physicians are reluctant to change, you also have a barrier. You'll want to recognize this concern and think of ways in which you will address it.

Exhibit 3.1 is a worksheet for the strategic portion of your business plan. It has places for your mission; vision; values; goal categories and goals; projects; barriers and opportunities; and strategies. This exhibit can also be found on the website www.radcliffe-oxford.com/medicalpracticemanagement.

EXHIBIT 3.1 Business plan worksheet

PRACTICE NAME – BUSINESS PLAN			
Mission			
Vision			
Values			
Goals	*Year 1 Projects*	*Year 3 Projects*	*Year 5 Projects*
Practice organization and management			
Quality and quality improvement			
Financial management			
Human resources			
Practice operations			
Compliance			

Year 1 Projects	Barriers	Opportunities	Strategies

Year 3 Projects	Barriers	Opportunities	Strategies

Year 5 Projects	Barriers	Opportunities	Strategies

The strategic portion of your business plan lays the foundation for your financial plan. In order to make the transition from strategy to finance, list your *assumptions*. For example, if your strategy is to open a satellite office to enlarge the service area for which you provide care, state your assumptions about the size and location of that office and projected opening date. When you do your financial forecasting, you can revisit your assumptions and make any changes that are needed. Likewise, if one of your strategies is to offer a new service, state your assumptions about the fees you will charge and start-up costs. Exhibit 3.2 contains some of the assumptions used for the development of the operating and capital budgets for a specialized pediatric practice.

EXHIBIT 3.2 Sample assumptions for practice operating and capital budgets: partial list of assumptions for operating and capital budgets

General information on the practice: The practice provides comprehensive testing to children and adolescents who have difficulties in learning. The clinical team includes pediatricians, psychologists, and learning specialists.

Volume projections
▶ The practice will gradually build up the volume of patients for whom the clinicians provide services. In year 1, 50% capacity in months 1–6; 75% capacity in months 7–12. In year 2, 75% capacity in months 1–3; 100% capacity in remaining months.
▶ The practice will provide three levels of care, each of which will be projected in the business plan: initial consultation at the practice; comprehensive full-day evaluation at the practice; and telephone follow-up.

Revenue projections
▶ Fees for each level of care are: initial consultation ($875); comprehensive testing ($2,500); follow-up ($100/hour).
▶ The practice will not file insurance claims with managed care plans and other payers. Therefore, there will be no contractual adjustments.
▶ Assumption about bad debt: 10% of patients will not pay on time.
▶ The practice will generate both operating revenue and grant revenue.

Operating expenses
▶ Annual inflation will be equal to the CPI.
▶ Staff training: $1,500/person/year for senior staff; $750/person/year for all others.
▶ Marketing: 2 newsletters/year @ $2,000 each; development of new brochures; creation of patient information packages.
▶ Mailing: newsletters will be sent by email to 75% of mailing list; remaining 25% will be sent through US Mail at bulk rate.
▶ Consultants: marketing ($5,000), information technology ($15,000).
▶ Professional services: legal ($10,000), accountant ($7,500).

Capital expenses
▶ For year 1, all furniture will be borrowed from another clinic. Purchase will occur in Month 1 of Year 2.

The next part of your financial plan is your *operating budget*. Here's where you identify volume, operating revenue, and operating expenses. If you are just getting started, you'll want to use your best judgment, since you can't rely on historical information. If you are already in practice, project the volume for existing services by looking at historical trends and by factoring in any changes that you expect to occur. For example, if you have recruited an additional physician, make sure to project the volume for him/her; it won't show up in last year's figures. When you project volume for new services, be realistic. More than one practice has confused hope for great success with reality and then developed misleading and unattainable volume projections.

To project operating revenue, look both at historical information and revenues you expect to generate from new services. If you anticipate any significant changes in reimbursement from public and/or private payers, incorporate them here. Make sure to distinguish between your charges (i.e., gross revenue) and the amount that the payers will actually reimburse. You know only too well that in healthcare, gross and net revenue are two different numbers. For operating expenses, look at historical data and future plans. Be sure to include a realistic inflation factor. Exhibit 3.3 can be found on the website www.radcliffe-oxford. com/medicalpracticemanagement and contains a sample operating budget.

After you have developed your operating budget, develop a *capital budget*. You have four options for evaluating capital investments. Two satisfy the long-range decision rule and two do not. Exhibit 3.4 contains helpful information. A good source of additional information is Ernest J Pavlock's *Financial Management for Medical Groups*.[1]

EXHIBIT 3.4 Techniques for capital budgeting

TECHNIQUE	SATISFIES LONG-RANGE DECISION RULE
Net present value method	Yes
Internal rate of return method	Yes
Payback period method	No
Average rate of return method (or unadjusted rate of return method)	No

Next, bring all of your financial information together into a cash flow statement and balance sheet. The information that you place on these two sheets will help you determine whether or not you can afford to do what you want to do when you want to do it, or if you should go back and change your assumptions. It will also help you determine whether or not you need financing for any of your projects. Exhibit 3.5 contains a sample balance sheet and can be found on the website www.radcliffe-oxford.com/medicalpracticemanagement.

Once you have completed the strategic and financial components of your business plan, you are ready to move on to the third and final component, the implementation plan. Here's where you list the specific *action steps* you will take along with specific responsibilities and timelines. For example, if you know you want to add clinical capacity to your practice by recruiting additional physicians, specific action steps might be agreement on the specialty area that you wish to enhance, identification of the professional and personal characteristics of the type of physician that you want to bring into the practice, conversion of this information into a formal job description, contacting physician recruitment firms and appropriate training programs, placing an ad, identifying three potential candidates, interviewing candidates, checking references, making your decision, extending and negotiating the offer, and integrating the terms of the arrangement into a legal document. You'll want to assign responsibility for each of these steps to one or more individuals and to specify a time frame.

How do you use your business plan after you complete it?

You can use your business plan in at least five ways: as a guide for decisions, as a checklist against which to measure progress, as a recruitment tool, as the basis for requesting financial support, and as a way to link individual job descriptions to the priorities of your practice.

First, use your business plan as a guide to help you make decisions. Depending on your values, you can strictly adhere to the plan or use it as a flexible guide. In either case, refer back to it each and every time you make an important decision. If someone in your practice generates an idea that appears to make sense, compare the idea with your plan and test it for consistency. You can deviate from your plan as long as you realize what you are doing and that you may need to sacrifice something that is already in the plan.

Second, use your business plan as a checklist against which to measure your progress. Make it an important part of all of your meetings, remembering to reinforce its role as the roadmap for your practice.

Third, use the business plan as a recruitment tool. When you recruit and hire new physicians and/or staff, let your plan tell your story. To an outsider, the very fact that you have a plan can be a powerful characteristic that distinguishes you from other, less focused practices.

Fourth, use the plan to obtain financial support if you need it. Your banker will be pleased to know that you have carefully planned the project for which you are requesting support.

Fifth, use the plan to make sure that the job descriptions for individuals within your practice are consistent with your practice's stated goals.

Who should participate in the planning process?

The process of developing a business plan is as important as the content, so pay careful attention to the process that you use and the people whom you involve. Seek input from inside and outside your practice.

Within your practice, designate one individual to lead the development of your business plan. If you are just starting out in practice, you may be both the leader and the entire team. That's fine; as you grow and repeat the planning process, you can add participants. If you are an existing practice, involve every partner and staff member in the process in some way. If your practice employs more than 15 people, consider designating a business planning task force that represents your physicians, nurses, front office, back office, and other areas of your practice.

Individuals outside your practice can enhance your business planning process in several ways. A general practice management consultant can provide guidance in collecting and organizing information about your practice and about the environment in which you function. This same consultant can objectively facilitate a planning retreat.

Other people outside your practice who can provide input are your accountant and attorney. Once you have determined the strategic portion of your plan, your accountant can run the numbers. Your attorney can inform you of any anticipated changes in laws and regulations that will impact your practice.

Be sure to talk with representatives of the hospital(s) and other healthcare facilities to which you admit patients. Ask about long-range plans so you are aware of opportunities that may benefit your practice. If you are part of an IPA, PHO, or other collaborative organization, check with them as well.

Finally, go outside your immediate community and solicit input from your state and local medical societies and hospital associations. The more data you have on the healthcare environment, the better off you will be.

When should you develop a business plan?

If you are just starting out in practice, developing a business plan before you open your doors will help you clarify your thinking about your practice. Your first business plan does not have to be perfect, and you should expect to revise it within a year.

If you are already in practice, develop a three- to five-year business plan with specific goals for the coming year. Use the plan during the year to monitor your progress. Revisit the plan in a year and make any necessary revisions. Within three to five years, develop another plan. You are already familiar with the business planning process and should easily be able to update much of the information you already collected for your first plan.

You should also create a business plan for every new service or revenue stream that your practice considers in the future. The same logical process that drives the practice's overriding direction also applies to individual investments. For example, expanding at your current site, relocating to a new location, adding new services, or purchasing the real estate that the practice currently leases are all situations that require a formal business plan.

What steps should you take – and in what order?

The process of developing a business plan for your practice has seven steps. They are listed in the order in which you should take them. If you are just starting out in practice and are not involving many physicians and staff, modify these steps accordingly.

Establish direction and leadership

1 Designate an individual in your practice to lead your business planning process.
2 Develop your business planning team, making sure to include clinical and administrative representatives of your practice.
3 Identify at least two external consultants that can help you collect information and facilitate your business planning retreat. Meet with both consultants, request proposals, check references, and select one.
4 Communicate your business planning process to everyone in your practice and explain what role each person will play.

Gather information

5 With the consultants, develop a list of questions that you want to answer about the healthcare environment and about your practice. Appendix B contains a comprehensive list of questions for which you need answers and can be found on the website www.radcliffe-oxford.com/medicalpracticemanagement.
6 Collect information from within your practice and from outside sources. One-on-one interviews within your practice work well.
7 Obtain input from your accountant, your attorney, and other external consultants.
8 Organize the information that you have gathered so that it can be used as input for your planning retreat.

Hold a planning retreat

9 Plan your planning retreat.
10 Hold your retreat, preferably offsite to minimize distractions for the participants.
11 During the retreat, create the strategic component of your business plan.
12 Following the retreat, review the strategic component of your plan with everyone in your practice.

Develop your financial plan

13 With your accountant, develop the assumptions and financial spreadsheets that support your strategic plan.
14 Determine whether or not you can afford your strategic plan.
15 Revise the strategic plan/financial plan until you are comfortable with both.

Develop an implementation plan

Your implementation plan should specify responsibilities as well as time frames.

Share your plan

Share your entire plan with your practice and with the external consultants who have assisted you.

Use your plan

Use your business plan as a guide on an ongoing basis

What are the keys to a successful business planning process?

As you go through the business planning process, keep in mind the importance of these key factors: simplicity, good assumptions, relating financial resources to strategic plans, participation, leadership, collection of good information, careful planning for your retreat, and motivating and rewarding staff.

▶ *Simplicity:* Establish a clear business planning process, and make sure that the information you present to the participants in your process is clear. Use diagrams, stories, and examples. Remember that people learn in different ways. Some prefer reading, and others learn better by listening or watching a visual presentation.

▶ *Make good assumptions:* The financial plan that supports the strategic portion of your business plan is only as good as your assumptions. Spend time on the assumptions, not on the generation of spreadsheets.

▶ *Relate financial resources to strategic plans:* Believe it or not, many practices jump right into the financial portions of their plans without clarifying the strategy. Both are essential, so put the horse before the cart.

▶ *Participation:* If you are an established practice, participation by all physicians and staff will generate good ideas and opinions and help with acceptance. Emphasize the importance of every participant's point of view, and make sure your facilitator involves everyone in the process.

▶ *Leadership:* Your business planning process has multiple steps, so you'll need a good leader to provide guidance for your practice and for the external consultants with whom you work.

▶ *Collect good information:* The development of a business plan gives you the opportunity to collect information from within and outside your practice. It's all there; you just need to determine how to obtain and display it.

▶ *Carefully plan your retreat:* If you are convening an offsite retreat, plan it carefully. Make the event a participatory exercise. Encourage participants to get to know each other socially.

▶ *Motivate and reward staff:* Some of the participants in your business planning process may have participated in a similar process in another practice or as a member of a community organization. For many participants, however, the experience will be new and overwhelming. Take time to explain, motivate, and say thank you.

What are common challenges to successful business planning and how can you overcome them?

There are at least four challenges to successful business planning: failure to appreciate the importance of planning, lack of leadership, unwillingness to look honestly at your practice, and resistance to change.

The single greatest challenge for most practices is acknowledging that business planning is essential for the entity's future well-being. Hopefully, the preceding discussion addresses this concern.

New initiatives require leadership. Although there are entire libraries of books on the topics of organizational leadership and team building, physicians do not always read what is available. Without leadership, business planning fails. Leadership helps a practice establish a structure for decision-making. The leader helps to maintain focus and guide the processes of business decisions. The leadership role can be entrusted to a physician on a full-time basis or rotated among peers, depending on the physicians' interest and skill level.

A third challenge to successful business planning is unwillingness to look honestly at the current status of the practice. Physicians are generally more comfortable assessing clinical data and outcomes than they are applying critical thinking to the business of managing a medical practice. They find it hard to acknowledge that the practice of medicine is a service business, where customer needs and efficient, effective, and reliable service delivery really matter. Paying attention to market perceptions of your medical practice doesn't demean the clinical practice of medicine; it simply adds another dimension.

Finally, the development of a business plan for your practice requires a commitment to change. Many people fear change, and physicians are no exception. A business plan can create new opportunities for physicians to improve the quality of life and practice profitability while enhancing the quality of care for patients.

References

1   Pavlock EJ. *Financial Management for Medical Groups.* Englewood, CO: MGMA; 2000.

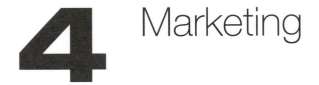

Marketing

The marketing of your medical practice will have a direct impact on your ability to satisfy and retain current patients and attract new ones. Every clinical and administrative aspect of what you do, including patient care, governance and management, financial management, human resources, quality improvement, and practice operations will play a role. This chapter answers the following questions:

▶ What is marketing and why should your practice develop a marketing program?

▶ What are the attributes of an effective marketing program?

▶ Toward which individuals and groups of people should you market your practice?

▶ What marketing techniques should you use?

▶ How can you use a practice website to enhance your value to patients?

▶ How can you measure the effectiveness of your marketing program?

▶ What types of external experts can help you with your marketing program?

▶ What legal and ethical constraints impact marketing in your practice?

What is Marketing and Why Should Your Practice Develop a Marketing Program?

The well-known management consultant Peter Drucker called marketing your "whole firm, taken from the customer's point of view." Taken one step farther, marketing means "your coordinated efforts to communicate with and persuade customers to purchase, use, and repurchase the services you provide through multiple points of influence".[1] The American Medical Association offers another definition. It's the process of planning and executing the conception, pricing, promotion, and distribution of ideas, goods, and services to create exchanges that satisfy individual and organizational objectives.[2]

You should market your practice for at least three reasons. First, you are in a competitive situation, like it or not. Second, although patients themselves make decisions about which physician to see, they also rely heavily on the influence of others. You want both patients and influencers to know about your practice. Third, although you may prefer to believe that patients come to your practice because of your clinical excellence, remember that they judge many other features of your practice such as the location, parking, customer service, technology, and reputation.

Competition

Unless your practice is located in an area with a physician shortage in your specialty, you have competition. The newspapers, Internet, and radio and television bombard people with information about medical care whether they want it or not. Patients and medical colleagues who refer to you know they have choices about where they respectively seek medical care and refer patients. If you don't remind both groups about the clinical and administrative advantages of your practice, they may go elsewhere. If you are proud of the patient care that you provide and the ways in which you do it, say so!

Role of Influencers in Healthcare Decision-Making

Healthcare is different from other sectors of the economy. Patients do make choices about physicians and facilities, but they actively seek out and rely on the advice of others. They ask their family, friends, and neighbors for recommendations. If these influencers have had a positive experience with your medical practice, they will spread the good word. If they have had a negative experience, they will spread that negative word too – faster and farther.

Other important influencers of patient decisions are physicians and health plans. Although primary care physicians no longer function as gatekeepers with the frequency that they did in the 1980s and 1990s, they remain in a unique position to refer patients to medical and surgical specialists when the need arises. Managed care plans influence patients too. Most plans give patients financial incentives to seek care from in-network physicians, and so if you are not part of those networks, you may lose patients to other physicians. The connection between referring physicians and managed care networks is also important. If physicians who can refer patients to you learn that you are not a network provider for a particular managed care plan, they may find it easier not to send you any patients at all rather than to remember the networks in which you participate.

How Patients Judge Your Practice

Finally, in this age of consumer supremacy, patients want good clinical care combined with administrative efficiency. They judge the total experience. They care about the ease of making appointments, checking in at your front desk, ordering prescription refills, and obtaining test results. They expect respectful interactions with your billing and collections staff. If they are satisfied with their clinical care but dissatisfied with the administrative aspects of your practice, they might look for a new physician in a different practice. Exhibit 4.1 describes Ms Nicholas, a patient who is considering changing her primary care physician.

EXHIBIT 4.1 Ms Nicholas' frustrations with her primary care physician

Ms Nicholas is a healthy and active 60-year-old woman living in a university town in a southern community. Her primary care physician is part of a ten-person private practice, and her gynecologist is on the staff of the academic medical center in town. Ms Nicholas rarely contacts her primary care physician because of the many administrative barriers to what she considers to be good patient care. If she calls to make an appointment or to ask a question, she talks with an operator, never with a physician or nurse. The operator relays a detailed message to a nurse who calls back to ask the same questions that the operator just asked. When Ms Nicholas schedules an office visit, she repeats that same information two more times before her physician actually talks with her about her symptoms, a diagnosis, and a treatment plan. If the physician orders tests, Ms Nicholas receives them only if she calls again and speaks to multiple people. It's a frustrating process – so frustrating that Ms Nicholas is seriously considering changing her primary care physician to a different internist who practices in a more patient-friendly practice. In contrast, when Ms Nicholas contacts her gynecologist, an automatic answering machine takes the message, and a triage nurse calls back immediately. Once that nurse has the information, Ms Nicholas does not need to repeat it multiple times. She makes an appointment, and at the time of her visit the physician verifies the information that was collected ahead of time.

Don't be like Ms Nicholas' primary care physician and neglect the importance of marketing. Actively market your practice – all the time.

What Are the Attributes of an Effective Marketing Program?

As you develop a marketing program for your practice, emphasize the seven attributes of an effective marketing program. First, develop a marketing program that is consistent with your business plan. Second, keep your marketing plan simple and specific. Third, make sure that everyone in your practice understands and supports your marketing philosophy and his/her role in implementation. Fourth, make sure your marketing efforts are measurable. Fifth, set attainable marketing goals so you achieve success. Sixth, make your program rewarding for your target market, you as a physician, your practice, your staff, and for your suppliers. Finally, make your marketing program timely.[3]

Relationship of Your Marketing Program to Your Business Plan

If you developed a business plan before you turned your attention to marketing, you have already reached a consensus within your practice on your mission, vision, values, goals, objectives, strategies, and action steps. Your marketing program is one way in which you can implement various aspects of your business plan.

Here's an example. Supposing you are an orthopedic surgery practice that has decided to offer physical therapy services at your practice site as a clinical enhancement and as a convenience to your patients. Just making the decision to add a service won't guarantee new business. You'll want to tell patients, referring physicians, and managed care plans the details of your new program so they understand how it can work to their advantage.

Simplicity and Specificity

Keep your marketing plan simple and specific. You want your entire workforce to understand and support it, and you want to use your plan to monitor your progress.

Here's an example from the marketing campaign by a foot and ankle center.[2] The same type of straightforward program can be used for most practices.

- Create a visual (i.e., graphic) identity with a logo and a tag line.
- Create an informational identity.
- Create an awareness of the foot and ankle center with current and potential patients.
- Provide foot and ankle patient education using a patient handbook and fact sheets.

▶ Place educational articles in local magazines and company newsletters.

▶ Develop an informational kit to leave with referring physicians.

Workforce Support

If you agree that everything you do in your practice is marketing, your entire workforce should be well-informed and actively supportive of your marketing program. You are cultivating workforce loyalty. Some people will of course play a more direct role than others in the development of your marketing material, but every single person should be clear about your practice's marketing philosophy, the different components of your program, and the role that he/she plays. Each workforce member is an ambassador for your practice, just as every employee of Disneyworld is an ambassador for a theme park that excels in guest relations.

Here's an example of the way in which one practice involves its employees in its marketing program. Nice Face Solutions in Merion, AZ has two physicians who specialize in cosmetic dermatology and facial plastic and reconstructive head and neck surgery respectively. The practice has two full-time patient coordinators whose job responsibilities include providing new patients with a practice welcome packet, making sure that new patient information is complete, providing an initial consultation for patients, and educating patients about the full menu of services that the practice provides. Most insurance companies don't cover cosmetic services, so patients expect to pay out of their own pocket for the services they receive. When the practice first started, it engaged an external marketing firm to manage its marketing program. It has become clear over time that the knowledgeable and enthusiastic employees, particularly the patient coordinators, can do a much more effective job.

Measurable

Your marketing program should be measurable so you know whether or not your efforts succeed. Keep careful track of how your patients heard about your practice. The information will help you understand the effectiveness of your different marketing techniques. One of the best ways to measure what you do is with satisfaction surveys for patients and for referring physicians.

Attainability

Make your marketing program attainable. Set realistic goals so you can successfully achieve your goals. If you have an ambitious plan with multiple steps, divide it into small sections. You don't have to do everything at the same time, but you do want each step to succeed.

Here's an example. A pediatric practice with two full-time and one part-time pediatrician developed a marketing program with 14 projects. They could accomplish some but not all of the steps easily. For example, revision of the patient brochure took two weeks, but development of a Personnel Manual required several months. The practice laid out a reasonable timetable that allowed it to complete these projects within a 15-month period.

Rewarding

A rewarding marketing program brings benefit to different groups – to you as a physician, to your practice, to your staff, to your referring physicians, and to your suppliers. Keep each of these groups in mind as you create and implement your program, and be sure to share the results with each of them.

Timely

Finally, your program should be timely. Give careful thought to the time of the year that you roll out your marketing program. Communicate your message at times when people are most receptive. For example, if you promote services directed toward nutrition and obesity, do so when people normally make fresh starts – i.e., when school starts, after the December holidays, or in the spring. If you schedule your program at holiday times, people are likely to be preoccupied with family events and not very interested in changing their eating patterns. Likewise, if you are a pediatric practice that would like to promote camp physicals, plan the program during the winter and implement it in the spring. Exhibit 4.2 describes the timely opening of a pediatric specialty clinic.

EXHIBIT 4.2 The timely opening of the student success center

The Student Success Center (SSC) is the clinical arm of All Kinds of Minds, a not-for-profit organization in Chapel Hill, North Carolina that offers multiple programs for students with difficulty learning. The well-publicized ribbon-cutting ceremony was deliberately timed to correspond with the opening of the school year, when parents, teachers, and students themselves were thinking about children and adolescents with problems in the classroom. Many months prior to the event, the SSC staff hired and trained staff, developed and tested operational processes, and announced the event through the media. The event took place on a beautiful fall afternoon, and the timing was perfect.

Toward Which Individuals and Groups of People Should You Market Your Practice, and What Techniques Can You Use?

An important aspect of your marketing program is the identification of the individuals and groups of people to whom you want to direct your efforts. Divide your target audiences into internal and external customers.[1] Exhibit 4.3 provides examples.

EXHIBIT 4.3 Internal and external target market groups

TARGET MARKET GROUP	SUGGESTED MARKETING STRATEGIES
Current patients	▶ Information package ▶ Newsletter ▶ Website bulletins ▶ Patient satisfaction surveys ▶ Birthday and/or holiday cards
Workforce	▶ Physicians – formal contracts ▶ Employees – personnel manual ▶ – performance evaluation program ▶ Entire workforce – clear understanding of their role in marketing

(continued)

TARGET MARKET GROUP	SUGGESTED MARKETING STRATEGIES
Potential new patients	▶ Brochure ▶ Website
Medical colleagues	▶ Thank you notes for referrals ▶ Satisfaction surveys ▶ Brochures, newsletters, website bulletins
Special demographic groups	▶ Educational information specific to the group
Local hospitals and other healthcare organizations	▶ Grand rounds and other programs ▶ Sponsorship of special events
Media	▶ Information on special services that you provide
Employers	▶ Assistance in providing employees and/or families with healthcare services that you provide
Health plans	▶ Special programs in your area of expertise
Local governments and public agencies	▶ Assistance in providing required services

Internal Marketing

There are two important target market groups within your practice: your current patients and your entire workforce.

Current Patients

Your current patients are already familiar with your practice. Make sure they are satisfied with your clinical care and administrative processes and continue seeking care from you. You want their loyalty. A comprehensive patient information package, consistent courtesy and good service from everyone in your workforce, and the opportunity to provide feedback through patient satisfaction surveys are three ways you can address this important target group. Consider a practice newsletter that includes information on your practice and on physician activities, testimonials from satisfied patients, and reliable educational material.

Here are three examples of messages you can direct toward current patients. With respect to clinical excellence, if you receive training in a state-of-the-art technique in your particular specialty, share your accomplishments with your current patients. If you introduce electronic health records into your practice, tell your patients that you are upgrading your practice in order to improve services for them and engage them in the change. If you develop a website that allows patients to use the Internet and your secure website to request appointments and/or pay bills, tell your current patients about the conveniences that you have added for their benefit. Promote your accomplishments and enhancements.

Entire Workforce

Your workforce can be your most supportive advocates or your worst enemies. They talk about you all the time to everyone they know, and if they are satisfied with the experiences they have on a day-to-day basis, they spread the word. Likewise, if they have major problems with the ways you care for patients and run your office, they spread that word too.

Your workforce cares about specific aspects of your practice. Your physicians expect good working conditions, including but not limited to the staff and office processes that support them, their compensation package, their call schedule, and financial support for continuing education. If they are dissatisfied with any of these factors, they are likely to voice their feelings publicly. The clinical and administrative staff wants the patient flow process to go smoothly. They want clear expectations about their jobs, timely feedback on their work and acknowledgement of their contributions to your practice. You need written job descriptions, a formal performance evaluation program, and consistent application of your policies and procedures.

External Marketing

Direct your external marketing toward potential new patients, medical colleagues, special demographic groups, local hospitals and other healthcare providers, the media, area employers, and health plans.

Potential New Patients

New patients come to you for one of three reasons. They may be dissatisfied with care that they received in the past from another physician in your specialty and want a change. They may be coming for a second opinion with the intention of returning to their original physician. Or, they may be new in your community and in the process of selecting a physician for themselves and their families. Be sure to ask new patients how they heard about your practice, and ask them what is important to them. Tell them exactly how your practice works, give them a clear and comprehensive new patient information package, and make sure that they not only try you out but stay with you.

An effective way to market your practice to potential new patients is to participate in community activities that give you visibility with the types of patients that you want to attract. Nice Face Solutions referenced earlier in this chapter presents informational programs for the public at a nearby wellness center. The center's members already care enough about their health to have joined the center, and many are interested in learning how to take better care of their appearance.

Medical Colleagues

If you are a medical or surgical specialist, your colleagues in primary care and in other specialties are a major source of referrals. Make sure that your medical practice and individual physicians with particular areas of expertise are visible in your community. Take time to visit other practices and/or socialize with other physicians. Find opportunities to provide education about your particular specialty to other physicians. Now that hospitalists provide most of the inpatient care at many hospitals, the opportunities for informal and spontaneous physician interaction are shrinking. You should create opportunities to converse with your colleagues and tell them about what you are doing in your practice.

Here are examples of ways to market your practice to medical colleagues. Use the same newsletter that you send to patients to keep your colleagues informed about what is going on in your practice. If you provide a specialty service like asthma management, offer to educate physicians in other practices on what you are doing. When these practices need help managing their patients, they will either send the patients to you for a consultation or call you for advice. When colleagues refer patients to you, thank them with a handwritten note expressing your appreciation. Follow-up with a written or electronic report of the consult and a call to make sure that the referring physician has the information he/she needs. Each of these techniques can strengthen your relationship with the referring physician and generate more referrals.

Special Demographic Groups

You can target the services that you provide to specific niche groups such as executives, seniors, members of one or more managed care plans, and/or patients with a particular chronic disease.[2] You know better than anyone which of these groups are already or could be important to you. Consider organizing a special program. Exhibit 4.4 describes the way a family physician targeted his diabetic patients.

EXHIBIT 4.4 Targeting diabetic patients

Dr Franklin, a family physician in Durham, NC has expertise in caring for diabetic patients. The physician and his colleagues are part of a practice that is owned by a university medical center. Although the endocrinology department of the medical center has programs that concentrate on diabetic patients, its emphasis is on research. In order to introduce an emphasis on diabetic care into his practice, Dr Franklin hired a nurse practitioner to educate his diabetic patients on a one-on-one basis and in group settings. He has also signed up to participate in a national registry so he can benchmark data on his diabetic patients against that of other practices.

Local Hospitals and Other Providers of Healthcare Services

The local hospital(s), long-term care facilities, nursing homes, laboratories, physical therapy practices, and other healthcare providers are all potential referral sources for you. Investigate opportunities to share information about your practice.

For example, you can share your clinical expertise with colleagues at your local hospital by giving a grand rounds and/or special program. You can also sponsor special events. If there is an unmet need in the community in which you have expertise, encourage the hospital or other organization to develop a new program focused on that issue. Volunteer to be the medical consultant, and as the program becomes funded, work out a suitable financial arrangement.

Local Contacts in the Media

Your local newspapers, radio, and television frequently feature articles and programs on healthcare topics. If you are doing something in your practice that you think would be of interest to the general public, it's free marketing for you. Pay attention to the articles and informational programs that you see and hear. Identify ways in which you might be able to make a contribution and introduce yourself to the appropriate writers and/or producers. Remember, they are always looking for good stories.

Area Employers

Employers face the ongoing challenge of keeping the cost of healthcare for their employees at a reasonable level. Particularly, self-insured employers have flexibility in the healthcare programs that they offer to their workforce. If you provide the types of services that might be of interest to local employers, contact the appropriate person in the human resources or medical department.

Here's an example from a pediatric practice. Each spring, New Hope Pediatric Practice provides camp physicals for its patients. Since most of the parents work, the practice developed a camp physical program that would be more convenient for families and that could be marketed through a large local employer. The physicians approached the nurse of a large manufacturing company in their community. In a collaborative fashion, the practice and the company set up a program for camp physicals that was held two Saturdays in May. Many of the parents who brought their children for physicals decided to change pediatricians.

Health Plans

Health plans vary in their attention and approaches to chronic problems, but they all have one thing in common. If they can find a way to provide quality care to patients and lower the cost, they'll explore the opportunity. Exhibit 4.5 describes a special program developed by Red Cross Red Shield of Georgia.

EXHIBIT 4.5 Red Cross Red Shield of Georgia's special program for in-office gastrointestinal procedures

Red Cross Red Shield of Georgia was interested in supporting the provision of in-office gastrointestinal procedures. Provided patients were not high risk, the cost of providing the care within a medical office was less than it would be in a hospital or other outpatient facility. The plan developed standards for good quality care and asked interested practices to apply for participation. The plan then selected a limited number of providers that met its qualifications.

Local Governments and Other Public Agencies

You may be able to market your services to local governments and other public agencies. For example, your local school district or public colleges and universities may be interested in working with private practices to provide specific services to students. Exhibit 4.6 describes the way a pediatrician worked with a non-profit health education agency to communicate information about his practice to school-age children living near his office.

EXHIBIT 4.6 Dr Blue's communication with school-age children

Dr Blue was a pediatrician who bought his practice from an elderly physician who planned on retiring. Dr Blue wanted to market his practice to young families with children. He approached a well-known community organization that provided health education programs to school groups. In return for Dr Blue's financial contribution, the organization included his marketing material in the health kits it provided to children living in the zip codes that the doctor wanted to target. Dr Blue became a household name.

How Can You Use a Practice Website to Enhance Your Value to Patients?

A practice website should be an essential part of your marketing program. As consumers become more and more computer savvy, you'll want to make sure that you have a website that contains, at the very least, a description of your services, physicians, staff, location and directions, and methods for patients and others to contact your practice. As is explained in Chapter 12, you can add functionality to your website so you communicate with patients regarding pre-registration, online test results, pharmacy ordering and refills, online bill paying, and patient education. The very fact that you have a website sends a strong message to those who access it: you are practicing twenty-first century medicine.

How Can You Measure the Effectiveness of Your Marketing Program?

There are three good ways to measure the effectiveness of your marketing program. First, when patients come to your practice, ask them how they heard about you. Keep written documentation of your referral sources, and you will be able to determine the success of your marketing efforts.

A second way to measure effectiveness is to do a patient satisfaction survey on a regular basis. Ask your patients about their clinical and administrative interactions with your practice. See Appendix C, Exhibit C.1 on the website www.radcliffe-oxford.com/medicalpracticemanagement for an example.

Finally, do a satisfaction survey for referring physicians. Ask your colleagues if you are meeting their needs, and, if you aren't, get suggestions for improvement. When you send a survey to other physicians, be sure to attach information on your practice. See Appendix C, Exhibit C.2 on the website www.radcliffe-oxford.com/medicalpracticemanagement for an example.

How Can You Use External Expertise to Help You with Your Marketing Program?

Your marketing program should be professional, and you may want to seek help from outside experts as you formulate your thoughts and implement your plans. Some of the people who can provide help are: a general medical practice consultant with marketing experience, a consultant who specializes in marketing, a graphic artist who designs your identity piece (i.e., your logo, stationery, brochure, and website), and a website design specialist who designs a website to correspond to your identity piece. Exhibit 4.7 describes the approach of an ophthalmologist who opened a new practice.

EXHIBIT 4.7 Announcing Dr Lenz's arrival

Dr Lenz completed his residency and fellowship training in the northeast. After much research on demographic trends, he decided to open a practice in a fast-growing community south of Raleigh, NC. Because he and his wife came to town with no contacts in the medical community, they were completely dependent on their marketing program to spread the word. They engaged both a general practice management consultant and a graphic designer to help them develop their materials and direct them to the right target groups.

What Legal and Ethical Constraints Impact Marketing in Your Practice?

When you develop a marketing program for your practice, be mindful of both legal and ethical issues. Ask your attorney for specific information on relevant federal and state laws. Here are some general guidelines.

First, remember your first priority – your patients. You are first and foremost a patient advocate. Your primary responsibility is to do what is appropriate for your patients. Don't let your enthusiasm for marketing interfere with your integrity.[3]

Second, avoid conflicts of interest. If you have a fiduciary relationship with a pharmaceutical company or other commercial venture, state this relationship right up front.

Third, make sure your marketing and advertising is not "false" and "deceptive." For example, if you are doing a procedure that has a particular result in most but not all cases, don't exaggerate the certainty of the result in an inappropriate way. Telling patients that a procedure is "guaranteed to reverse the ageing process within eight days," for example, is risky unless you can substantiate the accuracy of the statement.

Fourth, be mindful of the Stark Law as you develop your marketing program. If you contract with an independent marketing company for assistance, the safe harbor provisions require that the arrangement meet specific criteria. The Office of Inspector General has specifically identified the practice of waiving Medicare and Medicaid coinsurance and deductibles for reasons other than financial hardship as an anti-kickback violation.

Fifth, the HIPAA Privacy Rule requires that you obtain written patient authorization to use or disclose protected health information (PHI) for activities and communications that are considered to be "marketing." Examples of activities that qualify as marketing under HIPAA are:

1 Selling or giving away lists of patients to third parties for their use and reuse. For example, a medical practice cannot sell names of pregnant women to baby formula manufacturers without authorization.
2 Receiving payment from a vendor for marketing a particular product to your practice's patients.
3 Asking patients to invest in such things as multi-level marketing or in a new office building.
4 Selling or giving away a list of patients to Business Associates or other vendors for independent marketing use. For example, you cannot disclose PHI to pharmaceutical companies for those companies' drug promotions without authorization.

Finally, as a rule of thumb, follow these general guidelines suggested in the comprehensive Aspen Publishers manual, *Medical Group Practice, Legal and Administrative Guide*:[4]

▶ Avoid exaggeration and advertise/market exactly what you offer.
▶ Emphasize what you provide, not what the public might want.
▶ Use clear language that is easily understandable by the public. For example, words like "urgicenter" have different meanings to different people.
▶ Try not to create unrealistic expectations.
▶ Avoid representing your practice as having "higher standards" than others. How can you prove it?

▶ Make sure you can fulfill all promises under all circumstances.

▶ Avoid including price information in your marketing material.

References

1   Ross A, Pavlock EJ, Williams SJ. *Ambulatory Care Management.* Third edition. Albany, NY: Delmar; 1998.

2   Reid MJ. Customer, Where Art Thou? Niche Marketing in the Healthcare Industry. Downloaded from www3.mgma.com/articles/index.cfm?fuseaction=detail.main&articleID=13455; 2005.

3   Aronoff GM. Successful Medical Marketing for Practice Survival. In: Silver JK. *The Business of Medicine.* Philadelphia: Hanley & Belfus, Inc.; 1998.

4   Eldridge J, Conner C. *Medical Group Practice, Legal and Administrative Guide.* New York: Aspen Publishers; 1999–2003.

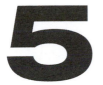 # Introduction to Financial Management

If you are a physician who is baffled by finances and uncomfortable talking about your knowledge gap, rest assured you are not alone. Many of your colleagues share your discomfort and hope that their practices will somehow survive and thrive without physician financial oversight. This chapter addresses the following questions:

- What does financial management of a medical practice involve?
- What concerns deter many physicians from mastering the financial management of their practices?
- How can you learn the basics of financial management?
- What information should you review and how often?
- To whom should you turn for advice when your financial oversight identifies problems?

What Does Financial Management of a Medical Practice Involve?

Financial management of a medical practice involves at least four different areas: budgeting, accounting, practice management (operations and clinical), and financial planning. A related topic, managed care, is included in Chapter 6 on Revenue Cycle Management.

Budgeting

In Chapter 3, you learned the importance of strategic business planning for your practice. An essential part of that planning process is the creation of a financial plan that supports your strategic plan. Your financial plan should include five-year forecasts, your plan for financing your practice, and an annual budget. That budget projects your volume, revenue, and expenses for a year. It becomes your tool for comparing your actual revenue and expenses against your expectations.

The steps for creating and using a budget are straightforward. Start with people and assumptions before you fill in numbers. First, establish a budget planning team that includes one or more physicians, your practice administrator/manager, supervisors as appropriate, and an external practice management consultant (optional). If you are just starting your practice, seek help from an external consultant.

Whether you are a new or existing practice, make a comprehensive list of assumptions that are likely to affect your projections. For example, external influences, rates of inflation, staffing changes, facility changes, and other factors will impact your volume, revenue, and expenses. Exhibit 5.1 contains a sample list of assumptions that Happy Face Pediatrics and Adolescents used for its budget planning. Happy Face has been in existence for several years; many of its assumptions reflect the practice's goal of improving its current financial situation.

EXHIBIT 5.1 Sample assumptions for budget planning for Happy Face Pediatrics and Adolescents

TOPIC	ASSUMPTION
Gross revenue	▸ The practice will revise its current fee schedule so gross charges represent a consistent percentage of the current year Medicare reimbursement. For CPT codes that Medicare does not reimburse, the practice will set fees.
Contractual adjustments	▸ The practice will renegotiate six managed care contracts to produce higher levels of reimbursement. ▸ If Yellow Cross Health Plan continues to be unwilling to negotiate for higher rates, the practice will terminate its relationship with this payer.
Revenue from health education	▸ In month 6, the practice will add a new service, health education. Since managed care companies often do not reimburse for this service, the practice will expect patients to pay an out-of-pocket cost.
Net collections	▸ The practice will change practice management systems, switching to a new ASP model vendor that has a financial incentive to maximize net collections.
Staffing/salaries	▸ The introduction of the new practice management system will enable the practice to eliminate 2.0 FTEs. ▸ Wages and salaries will increase by an average of 3%. The increases will occur on each employee's anniversary date. ▸ Senior staff members will be eligible for a total bonus of $10,000 to be divided among 3 people.
Employee benefits	▸ The practice will eliminate health insurance coverage for employee dependents.
Staff education	▸ As a cost-saving measure, the practice will reduce the annual education benefit for all mid- and entry-level staff to $100/year.
Telephone	▸ The practice will replace the current telephone system with a more efficient one.
Information technology	▸ Within 6 months after the change to a new practice management system, the practice will purchase an ASP model EHR system.
Insurance	▸ The practice will change insurance brokers in order to take advantage of more favorable premiums.
Travel	▸ Travel expenses will increase given the rise in gasoline prices.

After you have identified your assumptions, project your volume with as much detail as you can estimate. For example, if you are a primary care practice that depends primarily on office visits to generate patient revenue, use historical information to determine the percentage of office visits that will fall into different categories. Exhibit 5.2 provides the sample volume projections for Happy Face Pediatrics and Adolescents. The list of CPT codes in the far left column is a sample; it does not show the complete list of codes that this practice uses.

EXHIBIT 5.2 Sample volume projections for Happy Face Pediatrics and Adolescents

CPT CODE	LAST YEAR'S NUMBER OF VISITS	LAST YEAR'S % TOTAL VISITS	THIS YEAR'S NUMBER OF VISITS	THIS YEAR'S % TOTAL VISITS	NEXT YEAR'S PROJECTED VISITS
99201					
99202					
99203					
99204					
99205					
99211					
99212					
99213					
99214					
99215					
99241					
99242					
99243					
99244					
99245					
Other Codes					
All CPT Codes		100.0%		100.0%	

Next, list every CPT code that you expect to use and decide what fee you will charge. Many practices relate their charges to Medicare reimbursement rather than setting the fees at random. For example, if you are a primary care practice, you could set your fees between 150% and 200% Medicare. If you are a surgical practice, you could set them higher. Not all CPT codes have Medicare values. For those that don't, use your judgment to establish your fees.

EXHIBIT 5.3 Spreadsheet for estimating gross charges for Happy Face Pediatrics and Adolescents

CPT CODE	ESTIMATED VOLUME	YOUR FEES (130% MEDICARE)	ESTIMATED VOLUME X YOUR FEES = GROSS REVENUE
99381	10	135.01	1,350.10
99382	15	145.34	2,180.10
99383	20	142.39	2,847.80
99384	25	154.71	3,867.75
99385	30	154.71	4,641.30
Other CPT codes			5,700.70
All CPT codes			20,587.75

Now multiply your projected volume by your fees in order to estimate the gross charges that you will generate from patient care. Exhibit 5.3 provides a sample spreadsheet for estimating gross revenue. Once again, the list of codes is incomplete and is included here as a sample. This particular practice has been conservative in setting its fees; they are set at 130% Medicare.

The healthcare industry is unique in that the revenue you generate by multiplying volume by fees is heavily discounted. Most payers reimburse less than what you charge, so you need to estimate what is called a "contractual adjustment or contractual allowance" and deduct this amount from your gross patient revenue to arrive at your net patient revenue. You also need to deduct bad debts from your gross patient revenue.

Now that you have projected your volume and net patient revenue, create a budget planning worksheet showing volume, revenue, expenses, and net profit (loss) before physician compensation. If you aren't comfortable with your net income on your first attempt, readjust your assumptions until you are satisfied with the result. Exhibit D.1 in Appendix D contains a sample budget planning worksheet for a one-year period and can be found on the website www.radcliffe-oxford.com/medicalpracticemanagement.

When your budget is finished, share it with other members of your practice and obtain their approval.

In medical practices as in many other businesses, seasonal variations affect the distribution of both revenues and expenses over the months of the year. It makes more sense to compare each month or quarter with the same period from last year than it does to compare a month or quarter with the previous period of the same year. For example, if your practice offers flu vaccinations in October of each year, you should compare the October revenue and expenses of this year with those of last October, rather than with revenue and expenses from September.

Accounting

The accounting aspect of financial management involves documenting and reviewing what has actually happened in your practice. What activities (e.g., patient visits, procedures, surgeries, and diagnostic tests) have occurred as a result of the care that you and your colleagues have provided, and how have these activities translated into dollars for your practice?

Your accountant follows generally accepted accounting principles (GAAP) to produce three monthly reports for you: the income statement, the balance sheet, and the cash flow statement. Each of these reports provides dollar amounts and relates dollar amounts to time.

▶ The *income statement* shows revenue collected from patients and payers and expenses paid by the practice. The income statement may also be called the operating statement or the profit-and-loss (P&L) statement. With respect to time, the income statement tells you about revenue and expenses during a particular period of time. For example, Exhibit D.2 in Appendix D contains a sample income statement for the month of January 2006 and can be found on the website www.radcliffe-oxford.com/medicalpracticemanagement. Note that physician expenses are kept separate from other expenses so you can look at your practice operations separately from owner expenses.

When you review your income statement, look at four important numbers: total revenue, total expenses, expense ratio, and profit before physician compensation. Exhibit 5.4 provides additional guidance.

EXHIBIT 5.4 Suggestions for reviewing income statements

INDICATOR	COMMON OBSERVATIONS	POSSIBLE EXPLANATIONS
Total revenues	▸ Drops or increases in professional fees ▸ Fluctuations in patient refunds and/or allowables ▸ Collection problems	▸ Seasonal variations that occur regularly and are predictable ▸ Staff failure to handle refunds; renegotiation of managed care contracts ▸ Billing and collections staff failure to prioritize pursuit of accounts receivable by amount outstanding and date of service
Total expenses	▸ Unusually large expense	▸ Single large expense like payment of malpractice premium ▸ Catching up on past bills or paying in advance
Expense ratio (total revenue divided by non-physician expense)	▸ Changes in your ratio, suggesting a rise in overhead ratio	▸ Increase in cost of particular overhead items – e.g., fuel
Profit (before physician compensation)	▸ Variations in your practice's own profit over time	▸ Impact of one or more of the variations in revenue and/or expenses

▸ The *balance sheet* shows your financial position at the end of a particular point in time by listing your practice's assets, liabilities, and owners' equity. Most practices use a modified cash balance sheet (described below) so they can show items other than pure cash and recognize assets and liabilities that they expect to pay or receive within one year.

Exhibit D.3 in Appendix D, which can be found on the website www.radcliffe-oxford.com/medicalpracticemanagement, contains a sample balance sheet prepared on a modified cash basis. Current assets are cash, equipment, and prepaid expenses like quarterly or annual rent or malpractice premiums. Non-current assets are furniture, fixtures, and equipment, and accumulated depreciation such as real estate. Current liabilities are accounts payable, the principle of notes and loans payable within a year, and accrued payroll withholdings. Non-current liabilities are the principle of long-term notes payable.

▸ The *cash flow statement* summarizes sources and uses of funds. Cash generally comes into and moves out of your practice in relationship to three types of activities: operations, investments, and financing. The cash flow statement shows how much money came in and out of your practice during a particular time period. It helps determine your future cash flow potential, your ability to pay off your debts, and your ability to distribute cash to physicians. Work with your accountant to determine the most useful form of cash flow statement for managing your practice.

One of the most important issues about these three reports is time. You must understand both the difference between cash and accrual accounting and the modified cash accounting approach that most accountants use. First, with some exceptions, you don't receive the entire payment for care at the time of service. When you bill a public or private insurance company, there's a time lag between the date of service and the date when you receive the reimbursement. In any given month, then, your revenue "lags" behind your expenses, and it takes more than a month for the revenue to catch up to what you have spent.

The second time issue relates to how you record or "book" your revenue. Most medical practices use the cash method of accounting that records transactions only when cash changes hands. For example, when a patient or payer reimburses you, you record the payment on your books. Another method of accounting is called accrual accounting. With this method, you recognize the financial obligation at the time of service, and you record both revenue and expenses at that time. Still a third method of accounting is called modified cash accounting. This method follows the cash method and makes allowances for some non-cash transactions, allowing you to spread expenses over a period of time. For example, in modified cash accounting, you include on your balance sheet long-lived assets such as equipment over a certain amount and real estate, and assets and liabilities related to borrowing or investing cash (e.g., payroll withholdings and notes payable or receivable). Although you haven't written checks for these items, you are recognizing that they exist and then spreading them over time.

Practice Management (Operations and Clinical)

The third aspect of financial management concerns your practice operations and provision of clinical care to patients. In both of these activities, you must protect the dollars that you earn by managing and controlling overhead expenses and by developing and maintaining internal controls.

Managing and Controlling Overhead Expenses

The overhead costs of your practice are not connected with the production of goods or services. In a medical practice, then, these costs are those that are not directly connected with the provision of patient care. For example, your rent, or your depreciation if you own your building, are considered overhead costs.

According to industry standards, your overhead costs should represent somewhere between 45 and 60 percent of your total operating costs, depending on your specialty. MGMA's annual Cost Surveys are a good source of information. You can keep your overhead expenses at a desirable level by managing them in a very deliberate way. If overhead is higher than industry standards or higher than you would like it to be, your practice might suffer from one or more of the problems listed in Exhibit 5.5.

EXHIBIT 5.5 Common problems related to high overhead expenses

CHARACTERISTIC	POTENTIAL CORRECTIVE ACTION
Low patient volume	▶ If you close your practice at lunch time, consider seeing patients at this time. You are already paying your staff.
Outdated and inequitable fee schedules	▶ Review and update your current fee schedules.
Lack of administrative oversight of expenses	▶ Review the way in which you have divided administrative responsibilities for your practice and make sure you have accountability where you need it.
Inefficient staffing	▶ Make sure all job descriptions accurately reflect people's job responsibilities. ▶ Develop and use a formal performance evaluation system.

(*continued*)

CHARACTERISTIC	POTENTIAL CORRECTIVE ACTION
Higher than average staff turnover and recruitment expenses	▸ Make sure your wages and benefits are consistent with industry and community standards. ▸ Assist your supervisory employees to effectively manage those employees who report to them.
Managed care contracts that do not maximize the reimbursement for a practice of your size and specialty	▸ Renegotiate managed care contracts on a regular basis. Remember that payers don't come to you asking to pay you more; you must take the initiative.
Failure to develop operating and capital budgets and use them as guidelines for spending	▸ Use the instructions earlier in this chapter to create an operating budget. ▸ Develop a capital budget for your practice.
Lack of strategic planning	▸ Take the time to do a formal strategic plan and update it annually.

Overhead expenses that are too high are just one part of the problem. Your overheads might also be lower than standard for one or more of the reasons listed in Exhibit 5.6.

EXHIBIT 5.6 Common problems related to low overhead and expenses

CHARACTERISTIC	POTENTIAL CORRECTIVE ACTION
Inequitably high fees	Review your fees and set them at a reasonable level.
Patient care that falls below quality standards	Quality of care should be your #1 priority. If you are saving money but falling short of community standards, rethink your approach.
Understaffing	Consider staffing changes. Understaffing puts you at considerable risk for legal action.
Wages and benefits that are lower than community and/or industry standards	Compare the wages and benefits for your practice with industry standards in your region and make appropriate adjustments.

If your overhead expenses are either too high or low, you need to fix the problems. The American Medical Association offers many practical suggestions in its book *Financial Management of the Medical Practice*.[1] Exhibit 5.7 expands upon some of these ideas and can be found on the website www.radcliffe-oxford.com/medicalpracticemanagement.

Developing and Maintaining Internal Controls

In addition to managing and controlling overheads, make sure you develop and maintain internal control systems that help you manage the cash in your practice. Here are some practical suggestions:

▸ *Set up appropriate bank accounts:* Set up multiple accounts to help you manage your cash. The cash balance in your operating account should support your accounts payable and payroll. Don't keep any more here than you need to, since the money isn't earning interest. Set up a separate interest-bearing money market account for money that you don't need immediately, and transfer money from there to your operating account only when you need it. Finally, you can set up a separate payroll account, limiting access only to members of your practice who need to have it.

▸ *Manage your incoming cash carefully:* You'll be receiving cash, checks, and credit card payments from patients, from public and private payers, and from other sources. Exhibit 5.8 lists steps that you can take to manage your incoming cash.

EXHIBIT 5.8 Suggestions for managing incoming cash

SUGGESTED STEPS	COMMENT
Deposit collections daily.	Use daily deposit slips even if you skip a day and make two deposits on the same day.
Copy insurance remittance forms and attach Explanation of Benefits.	
Copy checks from patients and attach them to your daily collections summary.	
List each receivable separately on the deposit slip.	Facilitate checking back to see what you did.
Enter the check number for bulk checks.	If you have the check number, you can match a particular check to the EOB.
Manage your cash flow on a daily basis.	Keep track of beginning balance + daily deposits – daily disbursements = ending balance for the day.
Use historical information to identify trends.	
Pay your bills on a timely basis but not early unless there is a discount for early payment.	
Ask your bank for a working capital line of credit.	It's wise to have the protection in place if you fall short and need to borrow.

▶ *Manage petty cash:* By keeping a small amount in the fund, by limiting responsibility for the fund to one physician and/or the practice administrator/manager, by using numbered and signed "Received of Petty Cash" forms, by documenting all disbursements of petty cash, by making sure that the cash plus slips equals the predetermined amount of the fund, and by maintaining a detailed log. Other precautions you can take are requiring approval for all disbursements, not cashing employee checks from petty cash, and not providing employee advances from your petty cash fund.

▶ *Create internal checks and balances:* Designating "someone you trust enough" to handle all aspects of cash collections and deposits or to manage all parts of the patient account cycle (i.e., charges, payments, and adjustments) makes you vulnerable to unintentional error and fraud. Your accountant can help you determine formal processes that are appropriate for your practice.

▶ *Protect your practice from fraud by bonding:* Regardless of how carefully you recruit employees and perform background and reference checks, embezzlement is always a risk to your practice. Take the same precaution that groceries, department stores, and other retail establishments take by bonding all of your staff members. Bonding is insurance that will reimburse you for the amount of the embezzlement.

Financial Planning

Finally, you and your partners work hard. Protect your earnings by asking an experienced, certified, and reputable financial planner to assist you with financial planning for your practice. Chapter 9 on Outsourcing contains a helpful section on this topic.

What Concerns Deter Many Physicians from Mastering the Financial Management of their Practices?

The five concerns that often deter physicians from mastering the financial management of their practices are both common and addressable. These concerns are: presumption that somebody else is in charge, lack of leadership, information overload, limited reporting capability of some practice management systems, and lack of knowledge.

▶ *Presumption that somebody else is in charge:* It happens all the time – physicians presume that the accountant, the practice administrator/manager, or another physician is keeping a watchful eye on the financial management of the practice. These individuals may indeed be watching the finances of the practice, but perhaps not in an organized and coherent way that facilitates systematic information review, problem identification, and corrective action on a timely basis.

   Accountants often get the brunt of the blame: "Our practice is in financial difficulty because our accountant didn't identify our problems and fix them." Accountants record what has happened during a particular interval and at a particular point in time. They set up checks and balances within your practice to protect you against fraud. If you want your accountant to provide consulting assistance *and* he/she is qualified to do that, execute a separate agreement for consulting services that specifies the projects you want done.

▶ *Lack of leadership:* Many practices lack a clear physician leader who has the interest, drive, and skill to collaborate with the practice administrator/manager to monitor the current fiscal status of the practice and create a financial plan. One way to encourage a member of your group to take on a managerial role is to provide time and compensation.

▶ *Information overload:* Physicians often receive so much information that they don't know where to begin. The numbers may look interesting, but taken out of context and reviewed without a framework of understanding, they can be confusing and misleading. One way to prevent information overload is to ask your practice administrator/manager to develop a standard report package that you receive on a regular basis. A cover sheet that includes highlights can guide you through the supporting information.

▶ *Limited reporting capability of practice management systems:* There are striking differences among the reporting capabilities of the many practice management systems on the market. Some of the newer Application Service Provider (ASP) models offer reporting capabilities that are far superior to those of legacy systems. If you are either purchasing a new system or upgrading the product that you have, pay attention to this important feature. Avoid vendor relationships where the production of reports that should be standard adds costs to the amount you are already paying. Exhibit 5.9 describes the problems encountered by Valley Stream Urological Associates because of inadequate reporting.

EXHIBIT 5.9 Valley Stream Urological Associates' problems with accurate and timely reporting

Valley Stream Urological Associates was created when three small urological practices merged to create a single new group. The addition of several more physicians brought the total number of physicians to 11. Each of the small practices had outsourced its billing and collections to the same external vendor, and when the merger occurred, Valley Stream continued to use that vendor. Unfortunately for the practice, the billing and collections vendor used a practice management system that was unable to produce standard reports for its clients in an efficient and comprehensible way. The Valley Stream physicians and practice manager repeatedly requested information on their practice so they could understand their financial situation. They never received the information they requested, in large part because the practice management system vendor didn't have the appropriate software. Eventually, the practice made the decision to bring the billing and collections in-house and to contract with a vendor whose reporting capability was more in line with the practice's needs.

‣ *Lack of knowledge:* Although some physicians have business school as well as medical school training, most do not. For physicians who want to learn to manage their practices, there are many convenient ways to gain new knowledge. Seminars, texts, journals, CD-ROMs, and online classes are readily available. Be honest about your knowledge gaps, be proactive in your learning, and consider requesting help from an external consultant.

How Can You Learn the Basics of Financial Management?

If you would like to gain a basic understanding of financial management for medical practices, you can take as many of the following four steps as are appropriate for you:

1 Do basic reading about the financial management of medical practices.
2 Familiarize yourself with the vocabulary of financial management.
3 Enhance your knowledge by signing up for courses offered by professional organizations.
4 Ask a practice management consultant for assistance. He/she can give you a crash course in financial management for medical practices, including but not limited to accounting, practice operations, managed care, and revenue cycle management.

Appendix D, which can be found on the website www.radcliffe-oxford.com/medicalpractice management, contains the following learning aids:

‣ Samples of basic financial management forms (Exhibits D.1–D.3)

‣ Suggested reading material about financial management (Exhibit D.4)

‣ A list of organizations that offer courses on the financial management of medical practices (Exhibit D.5).

What Information Should You Review and How Often?

When you are ready to review information about your practice, what should you check and how often? Look not only at financial information, but also at other information that translates into dollars for your practice. If you develop a systematic review process, you will be more likely to identify problems on a timely basis than you will if you approach the review process haphazardly.

On a monthly basis, review information that gives you a complete financial profile of your practice. Your accountant is the best source of the three important financial reports, your income statement, balance sheet, and cash flow statement. Work with him/her and/or with your practice management consultant to format the information in a useful way. Some practices ask the accountant to add a cover sheet that summarizes important points for discussion.

Your practice administrator/manager should check your receivables daily. Who owes you money, how much do they owe, and how long have the invoices been outstanding? Your accountant's reports will give you total numbers, but not payer-specific details. This information is in your practice management system. If you or your practice administrator/manager are not comfortable extracting the reports that you need, ask the vendor and/or a practice management consultant for help. Hopefully once you explain what you want, you'll be able to access the information in a useful format without paying an additional charge.

On a monthly basis, review key ratios related to revenue cycle management. Chapter 6 describes the important ratios that help you understand your revenue cycle management and provides guidance for understanding what is going on with individual payers, particularly managed care companies.

Each quarter, use your patient demographic information to help you with marketing. Where do your patients live? Is the number of patients from specific zip codes that are important to your practice increasing or decreasing? If so, do you know why? Who among your medical colleagues refer the most patients to your practice? Are there physicians in the community that you would like to refer to your practice but who may not know anything about your practice?

What do patients and referring physicians say about you? Administer and review patient and physician satisfaction surveys quarterly so you know how you are perceived by the two groups on whom you depend for support. Make sure to correct any problems that you identify.

To Whom Should You Turn for Advice When Your Financial Oversight Identifies Problems?

If you learn to review financial information on your practice in a methodical and timely way, it won't take long for you to identify problems. Your next challenge is knowing what to do when you spot an issue. Who can help you understand what is going on and correct the problem? Start with your practice administrator/manager. He/she may have a good explanation for what appears to be a problem. Depending on the problem, you may decide to request external help from your attorney, accountant, and/or practice management consultant. Exhibit 5.10 provides some suggestions. Exhibit 5.11 describes the approach taken by Stonebrook Internal Medicine when it discovered major financial problems.

EXHIBIT 5.10 Correcting financial management problems when you identify them

PROBLEM	POTENTIAL SOLUTION
Monthly trend reports show alarming increase in expenses.	▶ Ask your practice manager about seasonal expenses. For example, if your malpractice premium is due in July, you can expect a large expense.
You experience continued high overhead expenses.	▶ Look carefully at the cause for the overtime. Is there really a need to do work after hours, or does a particular individual need extra money for personal reasons? ▶ Institute a policy that requires authorization for overtime. ▶ Make sure you are not paying employees who should be salaried (e.g., your practice manager) on an hourly basis.

(continued)

PROBLEM	POTENTIAL SOLUTION
The dollar value of your accounts receivable skyrockets out of control.	▸ Look carefully at the process that your collections staff (or external vendor) uses to work the accounts receivables. ▸ Talk with your billing supervisor or other staff member to better understand the process. You need priorities for pursuing receivables, policies for write-offs, and systems for documenting what staff members are doing on a daily basis.
You haven't added physicians, but expenses for continuing education are twice as high as last year.	▸ Agree on a policy for continuing education that applies to all physicians.
You discover discrepancies in your daily cash management.	▸ Immediately notify your attorney and accountant.
You sense that your revenue cycle isn't really managed.	▸ Seek help from an external practice management consultant.

EXHIBIT 5.11 Stonebrook Internal Medicine's solution to its discovery of major financial problems

Stonebrook Internal Medicine incorporated three years ago when a large primary care group with more than 65 physicians splintered into separate practices. Stonebrook had six physicians. At the time of its formation, Stonebrook set up an in-house billing and collections department under the supervision of its practice manager, who had previously been a human resources manager and wasn't particularly knowledgeable about financial management. Stonebrook also hired a member of the old clinic's billing department to manage day-to-day billing and collection functions. The practice manager and the billing supervisor were good friends who had always had an excellent working relationship. The physicians and the two staff members were confident about the success of the venture.

Several months after Stonebrook opened its practice, evidence of problems in the billing and collections department became apparent. Patients complained to their physicians that they were waiting too long for refunds or had received duplicate bills. Patients also claimed that they were not receiving EOBs from their insurers regarding visits to the practice, suggesting that Stonebrook had never submitted charges. When asked about these kinds of problems, the practice manager reassured the physicians that such glitches were typical parts of starting a new practice and would be resolved quickly. At this stage, the physicians were addressing many other issues and had faith in the judgment of their practice manager and billing supervisor.

Within six months, however, the physicians could not ignore the rate of collections. Revenue was much lower than had been expected, and accounts receivable were increasing at an alarming rate. The practice manager and billing department were working hard, but neither had an explanation for the collection problems. The physicians did not understand the billing and collections processes in depth, but they did begin to question the lack of experience of the practice manager and her close friendship with the billing and collections supervisor. Other staff members were intimidated and didn't speak candidly about the problems that they observed.

The physicians finally realized that nobody in the practice had the experience to diagnose and remedy the billing and collections problem. The Managing Partner contacted the former Executive Director of the larger clinic of which the practice had been a part and requested outside help. The ex-Executive Director spent an afternoon reviewing the performance of the billing and collections department and identified problems and solutions. Claims were being entered correctly, but processing of denials was inconsistent, and documentation on the status of particular claims was poor. The average number of days in accounts receivable was 130 – way above the industry average.

The Managing Partner of Stonebrook conveyed the bad news to the partnership. The billing and collections department was a disaster. With the help of an external consultant, the physicians concluded that staff inexperience, not fraud, was the problem. Stonebrook decided to outsource billing and collections to a reputable local vendor with many years' experience in billing for primary care practices. The vendor and the practice agreed on mutual goals and a reasonable time frame for correcting the problems.

References

1   The Coker Group. Stanley K (editor/project manager). *American Medical Association's Financial Management of the Medical Practice. The Physician's Handbook for Successful Budgeting, Forecasting & Cost Accounting.* Norcross, GA: Coker Publishing Company, LLC; 1996.

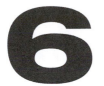 Revenue Cycle
Management

The financial health of your practice depends on the services that you provide to patients, the revenue that you generate from patient care, and your ability to collect exactly what each payer owes you on a timely basis. Revenue cycle management involves a series of related steps done collaboratively by multiple staff members. It is not a job for which one person is responsible. This chapter addresses the following questions:

- What steps should you take to develop a revenue cycle management program for your practice?

- Who should be responsible for your revenue cycle management program?

- What indicators and benchmarks should you use to monitor your revenue cycle management?

- What steps can you take to maximize patient revenue prior to the visit to your office?

- What strategies can you use to maximize your reimbursement from managed care companies?

- As the self-pay portion of your accounts receivable increases, what can you do to maximize the revenue that you collect directly from patients?

- How can you protect and enhance your revenue?

- How should you deal with your collection agency?

- How can information technology help you manage your revenue cycle management program?

- Where can you obtain help if you need it?

What Steps Should You Take to Develop a Revenue Cycle Management Program for your Practice?

Although the goal of maximizing patient revenue is common to all practices, the technique of achieving that goal using a revenue cycle management program is not universally understood. Particularly in practices without a professional practice administrator/manager, the term often elicits a blank stare that implies, "I don't even know what the term means, let alone have a formal program in place." Without a formal revenue cycle management program, staff members whose individual responsibilities impact the practice's financial health perform their responsibilities in isolation from each other without understanding how their particular jobs relate to the practice's overall ability to generate and collect revenue. Exhibit 6.1 describes a common scenario.

EXHIBIT 6.1 Short Hills Pulmonary Consultants' revenue cycle management program

Short Hills Pulmonary Consultants has five physicians. At one time, the practice contracted with a large national management services organization (MSO) that handled its financial management. When the physicians bought back their practice, they hired the MSO's former bookkeeper as their office manager. Neither the physicians nor the office manager understood revenue cycle management. They organized their new office in a way that separated the check-in and check-out functions from billing and collections. The front office people handling check-in were unaware that the accurate collection of demographic information and careful checking of insurance eligibility directly impacted billing and collections. The back office billing and collections staff did not set priorities and organize their work. On any given day, these billing and collections people made as many calls as possible with no regard to the amount and age of the outstanding invoices. The office manager was uncomfortable supervising, and so she didn't. The result was not surprising: more than $500,000 in accounts receivable accrued, much of it so old that the likelihood of collecting outstanding balances was negligible.

The first step in setting up a revenue cycle management program for your practice is to understand the entire process, listing each step that you need to take. Exhibit 6.2 provides suggestions. Pay particular attention to steps 2–5; they require that you have a good understanding of what you currently have in place. Don't rush to implement solutions before you know your current problems. Exhibit 6.2 can also be found on the website www. radcliffe-oxford.com/medicalpracticemanagement.

EXHIBIT 6.2 Suggested steps for revenue cycle management program

STEP #	DESCRIPTION	COMMENT
1	Create an internal revenue cycle management team and identify external resources that can contribute to the team's efforts.	Include on your internal team: physician(s), practice administrator/manager, representatives of front office, back office, coders, nursing, external billing and collections vendor (optional), and general practice management consultant (optional). Seek external help from your accountant and practice management system vendor.
2	Document and analyze current processes, highlighting systemic problems.	Be honest, not defensive in your analysis of work flow processes.
3	Use 7 indicators to measure the status of your accounts receivable and assess the effectiveness of your current managed care strategy.	Review indicators monthly to identify problems before they multiply and compound.
4	Use indicators to compare your practice with national and regional standards and take corrective action.	Use information from MGMA and other reliable professional organizations.

(continued)

STEP #	DESCRIPTION	COMMENT
5	Collect payer-specific information and identify problems.	Extract payer specific information from your practice management system. Seek help from your vendor if necessary.
6	Summarize the problems identified in steps 2, 3, and 4.	Combine the results from your observation of processes, calculation of standard ratios, and payer-specific information.
7	Develop and implement solutions to your problems.	
8	Measure the impact of your improvements.	
9	Renegotiate managed care contracts as appropriate.	Engage external consultant if your practice lacks internal expertise.
10	Document your revised approach to revenue cycle management, calculation of ratios, and payer-specific issues.	Reduce the risk of having key staff members leave without written documentation of all revenue cycle management processes.
11	Train your staff.	
12	Repeat the cycle.	Revenue cycle management never ends!

Who Should Be Responsible for Your Revenue Cycle Management Program?

The best way to develop and implement a comprehensive revenue cycle management program for your practice is to create both an internal team and an external advisory group. Your internal team should include one or more physicians, the practice administrator/manager, and representatives of your front office, back office, coders, and nursing. If you outsource billing and collections to an external vendor, include a representative from that company. If you would feel more comfortable with guidance from an external practice management consultant, seek help from someone recommended by your colleagues or by a reliable source like the state medical society.

Physician involvement is imperative. You own the practice, and one or more partners must retain oversight of revenue cycle management. Staff turnover in medical practices is notoriously high; people leave to pursue career advancement and for personal reasons. It is likely that physicians' longevity in your practice will be greater than that of your staff. Protect yourselves against the risk of not knowing how to generate claims or maximize the timely collection of revenue.

Your practice administrator/manager should play a key role in revenue cycle management. If your senior administrative person is a professional practice administrator, he/she should already have the knowledge and experience to develop, implement, and supervise your program. If, however, he/she is a practice or office manager, he or she may not have experience with revenue cycle management. Guidance from you and/or from an external practice management consultant can be helpful. Exhibit 6.3 describes the way a small otolaryngology practice introduced its practice manager to revenue cycle management and taught her to manage the process.

EXHIBIT 6.3 Beakman Ear, Nose, and Throat

Beakman Ear, Nose, and Throat was a small otolaryngology practice with three physicians and a hearing specialist. Following the departure of the practice manager, the physicians promoted a member of the billing and collections staff to take over her duties. Although the new practice manager had never run a medical practice, she was bright and willing to learn. An external practice management consultant taught the physician acting as managing partner how to formalize a revenue cycle management program, and he and the consultant shared the information with the new practice manager. With support and guidance, the practice manager took charge. She learned to extract indicators and payer-specific information from the practice management system, and she used the information to identify problems, find solutions, and monitor results.

Involve several people outside your practice in an advisory capacity. Your accountant, billing and collection/collection agency, your practice management system vendor, and a general practice management consultant can each be of assistance.

- Your accountant is a good source of historical information on your practice. The monthly income statements, balance sheets, and cash flow statements that he/she provides tell you what has happened in your practice. Request information for the past few years so you can review trends. Be mindful of the role of your accountant – to report on what has happened and to make sure that your business has the proper financial controls. Don't set unreasonable expectations for your accountant regarding problem identification and resolution. He/she is primarily a reporter; you are the fixer.

  Remember that revenue cycle management for medical practices is unique and different from that in other industries. Make sure that your accountant has experience with medical practices. Although familiarity can be comforting, choosing the personal accountant for one of the physicians as the accountant for the practice is unlikely to be sufficient in the long run.

- If you outsource billing and collection to an external vendor or use a collection agency, ask these parties for historical information on your practice.

- The information that you need to calculate important indicators should be readily available from your practice management system and your external billing and collections (or collections) vendor(s) if you have them. Some of the newer practice management systems automatically produce these reports for you. With some of the older systems, you may need to request and pay for customized reports.

- A general practice management consultant can help you better understand the entire revenue cycle management process and review the ways in which your practice handles each function.

What Indicators and Benchmarks Should You Use to Monitor your Revenue Cycle Management?

Seven standard indicators can help you monitor your current revenue cycle management. If you improve your revenue cycle management program, recalculate the indicators to measure the impact of your changes. The indicators are:

- Net charges to cash collections
- Net collection rate
- Gross collection rate
- Net days receivable outstanding
- Aged trial balance
- Bad debt
- Payer-specific information showing payment rate and actual vs expected reimbursement.

Net charges to cash collections: If you accept insurance, in most cases you will not receive reimbursement for the full amount that you bill (i.e., gross charges). The difference between your gross charges and what the payers reimburse is called your "contractual allowance," since you have agreed in your contracts to accept less than 100% of your charges. For this first indicator, start with your gross charges and then deduct the contractual allowances for each payer to determine your net charges. Your cash collections and your net charges should be parallel. Track them both on a monthly basis and monitor the trends. Your goal is to prevent cash collections from falling behind your net charges; you want them to be equal.

Net collection rate: Start with your gross charges and deduct the contractual allowance to get your net charges. Then compare your net receivables, the dollars that you actually collect minus any refunds or adjustments, with the net charges that you could have collected to obtain your net collection rate. This ratio is the vital sign for your practice's ability to collect revenue. Compare your ratio with national benchmarks and track your changes over time. If you identify problems, correct them right away. Older accounts receivable are the most difficult to collect.

Gross collection rate: Given the nature of your managed care contracts where the plans pay less than 100 percent of your charges, the gross collection rate is more of an indication of your contracts with payers than it is a barometer of the efficiency of your collections. If your gross collection rate drops over time when net collection rates remain stable, look carefully at payer-specific information on accounts receivable.

Net days receivable outstanding (NDRO) or days in accounts receivable: A good way to analyze the status of your accounts receivable is to divide your net receivables by the net charges/days in the period. (If you can't come up with the net receivables, use gross receivables.) This indicator shows you the average number of days that elapse between the date of service and the date when you receive payment. Compare your ratio with commonly accepted standards such as those used by MGMA to see if your practice is keeping up with industry norms. For example, well-run practices strive to keep their net days receivable outstanding at 35 or fewer days.

Aged trial balance: Another way to analyze your accounts receivable is to review the dollar amounts and the percentage of net receivables that are 30, 60, 90, and 120+ days old. If your analysis indicates that your 60, 90, and 120+ day old receivables are double digit percentages, you have a problem. Money that is 90 and 120+ days outstanding is the hardest to collect, and some practices automatically give these accounts to an external collections agency.

Bad debt: Next, compare your bad debt expense (write-off to bad debt less recoveries, not including charity care) with your gross revenue, and then compare information from your practice with the national average. If your bad debt is high, talk with your accountant about writing off some of the dollars. Then make sure you take corrective action so the problem does not recur.

Payer-specific information: The indicators described above can provide you with a general profile of your practice. They can alert you to systemic problems in your practice that can be corrected by improving your processes and assignment of responsibilities to staff. In many cases, however, you cannot identify and resolve problems without reviewing payer-specific information. Before you review payer-specific information, make sure that your practice management system and/or staff accurately reclassify dollars into appropriate categories. Ask yourself these four questions:

1 Do you reclassify to self-pay amounts that are not paid by insurance companies and that you are permitted to bill to patients?
2 Do you reclassify supplementary insurance (i.e., secondary payer) after the primary insurer has paid?
3 Do you separate dollars that patients are paying on instalment plans from self-pay accounts so you can monitor them separately? If you offer your patients payment plans, keep these dollars separate.
4 Do you re-age the dollars in self-pay after the insurance companies have reimbursed you? Affirmative answers to all four questions can help you obtain an accurate payer-specific profile.

When you are confident about the accuracy of your payer-specific information, create three spreadsheets. First, summarize general information about each payer so you know its importance to your practice (Exhibit 6.4). You want to know which payers represent the largest share of patients and dollars.

EXHIBIT 6.4 Sample payer summary for your practice

PAYER	# PATIENTS	# PATIENTS AS % TOTAL	GROSS CHARGES	GROSS CHARGES AS % TOTAL	NET CHARGES (GROSS CHARGES LESS CONTRACTUAL ALLOWANCE)	NET CHARGES AS % TOTAL
A						
B						
C						
D						
Medicare						
Medicaid						
Workmen's Compensation						
All Other						
All Payers		100.0%		100.0%		100.0%

After you know the importance of each payer to your practice, create a second spreadsheet that shows how quickly each payer reimburses you. In some cases, a single managed care company may offer multiple products with different payers, so check carefully. For example, Blue Cross Blue Shield of North Carolina offers its own managed care products and also provides administrative services only (ASO) for other plans such as the state employees. A meaningful examination of Blue Cross Blue Shield's rate of payment requires a separate analysis for the ASO products. Exhibit 6.5 contains a sample spreadsheet for displaying average payment rate for each payer.

EXHIBIT 6.5 Sample speed of reimbursement by payer

PAYER	% NET CHARGES	% ACCOUNTS RECEIVABLES	PAYMENT RATE
A1			
A2			
B			
C			
D			
Self-Pay			
Medicare			
Medicaid			
WC			
All Other			
All Payers	100.0%	100.0%	

Finally, just because you signed contracts with managed care companies doesn't guarantee that all payers abide by the terms of their agreements. Situations that frequently result in unintentional error may be the addition of a new physician in your practice or a change in the health plan's reimbursement level. Often the people in the health plan contract department negotiate new rates, but the operational people continue to pay at the old levels. Mistakes happen. Prepare a spreadsheet that compares what you actually receive with what the contract says you should receive (Exhibit 6.6). You may find that payment errors are costing you a lot of money.

EXHIBIT 6.6 Sample analysis of actual vs expected reimbursement for Somerset Family Medicine's managed care contracts

SOMERSET FAMILY MEDICINE REIMBURSEMENT ANALYSIS
PAYER NAME: MANAGED CARE PLAN A

CPT CODE	DESCRIPTION	EXPECTED REIMBURSEMENT	ACTUAL REIMBURSEMENT	DIFFERENCE (EXPECTED LESS ACTUAL)
10120	REMOVE FOREIGN BODY	110.00	106.00	4.00
12011	REPAIR SUPERFICIAL WOUND	146.00	126.00	20.00
ALL CPT CODES		256.00	232.00	24.00

What Steps Can You Take to Maximize Patient Revenue Prior to the Visit to Your Office?

Before patients come to your office, you can take at least four steps to improve your collections from both insurance companies and from patients themselves.

First, when a new patient calls to schedule a visit with your practice, collect demographic and insurance information before the actual visit. You can request the information over the phone by having one of your staff members talk directly with the patient. You can also mail or email a new patient information package and ask the patient to mail, email, or fax it back to you prior to the visit. Many practices post a new patient questionnaire directly on their websites so patients can fill it out at their convenience and send it back. Regardless of which approach you use, the goal is to obtain accurate demographic and insurance information prior to the visit so you can verify insurance eligibility.

Second, make sure you have written financial policies in place and that you share them with all new patients before their first visit. Be clear about your policies for no-shows, expected time of payment, and payment plans. Ask patients to acknowledge receipt of this information in writing. Exhibit E.1 in Appendix E lists the policies related to revenue cycle management that you should have. Appendix E can be found on the website www.radcliffe-oxford.com/medicalpracticemanagement. They fall into three categories: appointment scheduling, registration, and billing and collections policies. The Medical Group Management Association (MGMA) book *Operating Policies and Procedures Manual for Medical Practices*[1] contains the actual policies. Exhibit E.2 in Appendix E (on the website) contains a sample policy for No Shows, one of the most troublesome issues for many practices.

Third, if the physicians in your practice provide care for employees, for each other, and for physicians' families, determine your policies for charging for care and put those policies in writing. Most managed care companies have specific contract language that forbids you to waive charges for patients except under certain circumstances, so don't assume you can provide free care to special groups without risking payer reprisals.

Fourth, make sure your practice remains current on coding requirements for your specialty. When practices code below the appropriate visit level, they are leaving on the table money that is rightfully theirs. Both you and your staff can stay up-to-date by attending courses offered by your specialty society and by other professional associations.

What Strategies Can You Use to Maximize Your Reimbursement from Managed Care Companies?

Like it or not, reimbursement from managed care plans represents a large share of the revenue of most medical practices. Be proactive about negotiating the best rates that you can and about collecting what is owed to you on a timely basis.

Five strategies can help you maximize your reimbursement from managed care companies. First, establish good working relationships with payer representatives. Second, be well-informed about your current managed care contracts. Third, if you have the internal expertise to do so, develop systems for comparing reimbursement among the different plans and with local, regional, and/or national standards. Fourth, use the information that you collect on each payer to help you with your rate negotiations. Fifth, seek help from an external practice management consultant when you need it.

Establish Good Working Relationships with Payer Representatives

It is advisable to establish good working relationships with payer representatives before you discuss issues about reimbursement levels, claims problems, and information technology. Although you may refer to a payer as Payer A or Payer B, remember that within each payer organization, a team of people handles physician relationships. The person whom you call for operational questions is a provider relations representative; he/she does not handle the contract negotiation and claims resolution.

Once you know each plan's key people and their responsibilities, invite them to meet with you at your office. Share information on your current practice and your plans, highlighting anything about your practice that is unique and that might at some point justify an increase in reimbursement. Use the meeting to learn more about the payer. By creating good relationships with plan representatives, you can pave the way for more successful negotiations about rates when you are ready to talk about money.

Be Well-Informed

Although revenue from managed care contracts accounts for a large share of the revenue of many medical practices, there's an appalling dearth of knowledge about current contracts. Organize the general information that you already have about each plan using Exhibit 6.7 for guidance.

EXHIBIT 6.7 Sample managed care plan profile for St Nicholas Health Plan

---

Plan name: St Nicholas Health Plan

Contacts: (Names/titles, phone, fax, email)
  Jane Doe, VP Network Development
  John Stag, Manager, Contracting
  Jill Fawn, Director, Provider Relations

Date and term of current contract: Effective January 1, 2006 for 3 years

Current reimbursement rate(s): (% Medicare, fee schedule, or other)
  130% 2005 Medicare
  Plan fee schedule for codes not reimbursed by Medicare
  National fee schedule for lab codes

Operational issues in your practice: Inaccurate claims payment; 20% difference between actual and expected payment for the period January 1–December 31, 2005. Total amount owed to practice – $200,000.

Average rate of payment: (See previous section for instructions on calculating this ratio.)

Other information: Contract has not been renegotiated since 2002. Request higher rates.

Next, use your practice management system to create a payer-specific report showing historical volume and net charges for each CPT code that you have billed to the plan within the past year. Fill in the current reimbursement and calculate the net revenue that you should have received if the payer had abided by the terms of your contract. Exhibit 6.8 contains an example. Prepare a separate spreadsheet for each plan.

EXHIBIT 6.8 Sample managed care plan current reimbursement summary

SOMERSET FAMILY MEDICINE
NET REVENUE REIMBURSEMENT SUMMARY
01/01/04–12/31/05
PAYER: MANAGED CARE PAYER A

CPT CODE	DESCRIPTION	VOLUME (UNITS)	REIMB. AMT.	NET REVENUE (VOLUME X REIMB. AMT.)
10120	REMOVE FOREIGN BODY	25	98.00	2,450.00
12011	REPAIR SUPERFICIAL WOUND	110	146.00	16,060.00
ALL CPT CODES		135		18,510.00

Compare Reimbursement Among Different Plans and Against a National Standard

Once you know the total dollar value of patient care that you provide for each payer, ask two questions about the level of payment. First, is this payer paying you at the market rate of reimbursement compared to what you receive from other payers? Second, how does this payer's reimbursement compare with local, regional, and national standards? Surveys that you purchase from professional organizations may contain useful information.

Although the Medicare level of reimbursement has shortcomings, many practices use it as a baseline against which to compare the reimbursement level of different plans. Exhibit 6.9 contains two examples. For both CPT codes 10120 (Remove Foreign Body) and 12011 (Repair Superficial Wound) payer D is paying less than payers A, B, and C. Plan D is also paying less than Medicare.

EXHIBIT 6.9 Sample comparison of current reimbursement for managed care payers with Medicare

SOMERSET FAMILY MEDICINE
COMPARISON OF REIMBURSEMENT WITH 2005 MEDICARE RATES

PAYER	CPT CODE	DESCRIPTION	2005 MEDICARE	CURRENT REIMB.	CURRENT REIMB. AS % 2005 MEDICARE
A	10120	Remove foreign body	99.07	104.00	105%
B	10120	Remove foreign body	99.07	102.00	103%
C	10120	Remove foreign body	99.07	107.00	108%
D	10120	Remove foreign body	99.07	90.00	91%
A	12011	Repair superficial wound	144.72	158.00	100%
B	12011	Repair superficial wound	144.72	151.00	104%
C	12011	Repair superficial wound	144.72	158.00	109%
D	12011	Repair superficial wound	144.72	140.00	97%

If your comparison chart shows that different payers reimburse you at very different levels and that perhaps some of those levels are even lower than the current Medicare level of reimbursement, consider negotiating higher rates. Rather than pick a higher rate out of thin air, model the possibilities by starting with the current reimbursement as a percentage of 2005 (or current year) Medicare and by determining the impact on the bottom line of higher levels of payment.

Exhibit 6.10 contains a sample spreadsheet. Remember that from the payer perspective, what matters is the additional dollars that the payer will pay to your practice, not whether or not you think the reimbursement fairly compensates you for the care that you provide. In this particular example, the payer is paying Somerset Family Medicine $20,055.00 for the two CPT codes. If the reimbursement were to increase to 125% 2005 Medicare, the plan would pay $2,939.94 more, an increase of 14.6%. If the reimbursement were to increase to 130% 2005 Medicare, the plan would pay $3,859.74 more, an increase of 19.2%.

EXHIBIT 6.10 Sample plan modeling worksheet

SOMERSET FAMILY MEDICINE
REVENUE MODELING WORKSHEET

CPT CODE	DESCRIPTION	VOL.	CURRENT REIMB.	2005 MEDICARE RATE	REIMB. @ 125% OF MEDICARE	REIMB. @ 130% OF MEDICARE
10120	Remove foreign body	25	2,675.00	99.07	3,095.94	3,219.78
12011	Repair superficial wound	110	17,380.00	144.72	19,899.00	20,694.96
All CPT codes			20,055.00		22,994.94	23,914.74

The method for modeling different levels of reimbursement is a basic approach; it does not address every detail for every practice. Medicare doesn't reimburse all CPT codes, so your practice may be using important codes that cannot be analyzed in this way. Payers that reimburse as a percentage of Medicare may be using different years. Some payers use proprietary fee schedules that are not related to Medicare. Finally, this method does not use relative value units (RVUs) to analyze the cost of delivering care and then compare cost and reimbursement. Additional information on using RVUs for managed care contracting is available in the MGMA book *RVUs. Applications for Medical Practice Success.*[2]

Use Information that You Collect on Each Payer to Help You with Rate Negotiations

If you can make a strong argument justifying higher reimbursement from one or more payers, set up a meeting to discuss the possibility of a rate increase. If you've followed the steps suggested here, you already know the payer representative with whom you'll meet. Convene the meeting at your office. Describe the current status of your practice and your future plans, making sure to highlight the recruitment of additional physicians, the addition of new office sites, and the provision of particular procedures and/or services that may be unusual in your community. Indicate your willingness to sign a multi-year agreement if the payer will raise the reimbursement. Be persistent and professional, and you may be pleasantly surprised.

Many factors affect each payer's willingness or unwillingness to increase reimbursement rates. If you are a particularly important provider that is already providing care to many patients, the payer won't want you to drop out of its provider network. If you provide care to the employees of a large account that is important to the payer, the payer won't want to lose you. Depending on the way in which the payer is organized, there may be flexibility in the budget to provide an increase. It never hurts to ask!

Seek External Help When You Need It

Wouldn't you like to walk into a managed care negotiation with the same degree of confidence that you have when you enter an exam room to provide care for a patient? If you don't have the expertise that you need, ask an external practice management consultant to provide assistance. Chapter 9, Using Outsourcing Effectively, contains additional information.

What Steps Can You Take to Maximize the Amount You Receive Directly from Patients as Opposed to Insurance Companies and Other Payers?

The need for effective systems to collect directly from patients is growing in importance. If you accept insurance in your office, you should already be collecting co-payments and coinsurance at the time of the visit. But co-payments and coinsurance are just the beginning. As the cost of health insurance rises, many employers are shifting a larger percentage of the financial burden directly to their employees and offering Health Savings Accounts (HSAs). Your practice may decide to terminate your relationship with a particular payer and become an out-of-network provider. These kinds of situations have a direct impact on the dollars that fall into the self-pay category in your receivables.

Here are some suggestions for maximizing the amount you collect directly from patients.

Be tactful in patient communications: Let your patients know you value their business. Tell them that you may make financial decisions that require them to pay higher out-of-pocket costs. Be tactful. Avoid financial surprises for your patients at the time of their visits. If you terminate your relationship with a managed care payer, immediately send your patients a letter explaining your decision. Mention other provider networks in which you do participate and encourage your patients to remain with your practice. Exhibit 6.11 contains a sample letter written to patients by a practice that terminated its relationship with a major health insurance plan. Exhibit 6.11 can also be found on the website www.radcliffe-oxford.com/medicalpracticemanagement.

EXHIBIT 6.11 Sample letter to patients announcing health plan non-participation status

December 15, 2005

Earlier this month we sent you a letter alerting you to the possibility that our practice would no longer participate in Somerset Health Plan. We have been unable to reach an agreement with Somerset, and on January 1, 2006 we will no longer be network providers for the commercial or Medicare products.

As a valued patient of our practice, we want you to know that we did our best to reach a mutually satisfactory agreement with Somerset Health Plan. Our contract has expired, however, and we are now considered to be an "out-of-network provider." According to Somerset's rules, the patient portion of the bill for care is likely to increase.

We appreciate your business, and we would like to continue providing care for you and your family. If you keep Somerset Health Plan as your insurance, when you check in for your next visit, we will ask you to guarantee payment with a check or major credit card. If you decide to change your insurance carrier at the next opportunity, we will continue to participate in Powhatan, Truda, and Cedar Health Plans. If you receive your health insurance through your place of employment, you may also want to contact your human resources department and/or Somerset's Customer Service Department to discuss your concern with the situation.

Our practice regrets any inconvenience that our decision regarding Somerset Health Plan may cause for you. We will continue to provide high quality patient care and hope you will continue to support our practice.

If you have any questions prior to your visit, please contact Nicky Noodle, Billing Manager, at (215) 787-0223.

Sincerely,

Practice Name

Foster positive staff attitude: Encourage your staff to be assertive, not apologetic, about collecting money from patients. Good signage and careful staff training can ease the way. Convey the message that all patients are expected to pay their share of the bill, preferably at the time of service or within a reasonable time period following receipt of the invoice. You also want patients to know that you charge for no-shows.

Assure patient privacy: Set aside a private area where patients can discuss financial issues with your staff. Respect your patients' need for privacy and discretion, and don't put them in a long check-out line where other patients and staff can overhear their conversations about sensitive financial issues.

Provide ongoing staff training: Collections isn't a pleasant job, and it's easy for people to become discouraged. Help your staff to choose their words carefully so they can be brief, non-argumentative, intelligent, confident, businesslike, friendly, courteous, and flexible – and still get the money for you. Many practices script the words that they want their staff to use.

Meet with your collection staff regularly and give them the opportunity to talk about difficult cases. The art of collections lends itself to role-playing, and many practices use this approach to train their staff.

Turnover in the collections department is generally high, so offer refresher training on a regular basis. Don't assume that your new staff members understand the standards in your practice.

Help each staff member understand his/her role in relationship to that of other team members. Most people concentrate on their small piece of the process without a full understanding of the entire revenue cycle program.

Once you settle on a training program that works for you, document it so you can use it for future training.

Be sure that your staff know how to use your practice management system to its best advantage. If you are unsure about the availability of reports, contact your vendor.

Prioritize work: Help your staff prioritize their work according to the dollar amount and age of the claim. Encourage them to manage their time well rather than "making as many calls as they can" in between answering incoming calls. Their goal is to bring in the maximum amount of money, not spend time on the phone talking about relatively small claims.

Set productivity goals: Set productivity goals for both individual staff members and for teams of staff members if you have them. For example, a reasonable goal might be 70 telephone contacts per day (assuming 2.5 contacts per resolved account). Or you might assume that 1.0 FTE can resolve a certain number of accounts each month. Exhibit 6.12 contains examples of productivity goals for both individuals and for teams.

EXHIBIT 6.12 Sample productivity goals for individuals and teams in the billing and collections department

GOALS FOR INDIVIDUALS	GOALS FOR TEAMS
Highest dollar volume collected	Monthly cash goal
Greatest % increase in dollars collected	Dollar or % reduction in bad debt
Highest volume collected each day or week	Reduction in dollars that are 90+ days old

Monitor daily progress: In addition to setting productivity goals, ask your staff for regular collection reports. Review the accounts that your staff is working, each collector's ability to overcome obstacles, and his/her ability to obtain partial or full payment. If you monitor progress regularly, you can make helpful suggestions on a timely basis.

How Can You Protect and Enhance Your Revenue?

You can take many steps every day to protect and enhance your revenue. Here are suggestions. If you already have electronic health records (EHR) in your practice, that system may automatically eliminate most of the problems that are listed below.

Monitor your missing and late charges: Every day, run "missing ticket" reports to make sure that you have submitted all billable encounters to the appropriate payer. Overlooked charges add up. If your reports show patterns with particular staff members or physicians, remind them of the importance of submitting every encounter on a timely basis.

Match encounter forms with accompanying charges on a daily basis. Sometimes patients or staff forget to bring the appropriate paperwork to the checkout window. Check once or twice each day to make sure there are no missing charge tickets.

Review the encounter forms or screens that you currently use to ensure that you are capturing all the information that you need for billing. If the forms don't allow you to record payer-specific details, revise them. Your goal is to increase the percentage of "clean" claims that you send to payers.

Keep careful track of all hospital encounters and make sure to bill each one appropriately. Each hospital has its own system for notifying physician offices of admissions and consultations, so make sure that every hospital(s) to which you admit gives you faxed, hard, and electronic copies of encounter forms on a timely basis. Your practice management system may have a helpful function. If not, maintain a log that reconciles each physician's schedule with the hospital notification of charges.

How Should You Deal with Your Collection Agency?

Many practices engage the services of an external collection agency to help them pursue accounts that are more than 90 days old. This approach can be very effective if structured carefully. Here are suggestions for getting the best results from your collection agency. They address formal policies, paying for services, communication, and annual auditing and regular monitoring.

Formal policies: Develop a formal policy that governs the way your collection agency acts as your agent. Provide clear guidance and regular feedback. You, not your collection agency, should set rules and time frames for sending accounts to collections, for sending dunning letters to patients, for making follow-up calls, for writing off accounts, and for sending accounts out for legal action. You should have the final say on the wording of all letters that go to patients.

Paying for service: Most practices pay their external collection agency on a contingency basis related to the rate of recovery. If there is no collection, there is no charge to you. You can build a financial incentive into your rates and reward your collection agency for achieving benchmarks or exceeding expectations. Likewise, you can build in a penalty for not meeting the recovery rates on which you have mutually agreed. Many agencies are willing to reduce their rates for earlier placements, so investigate the possibility of turning over accounts to collections sooner than you currently do.

Communication: If you are doing some collections in-house and at a certain point sending accounts to an outside agency, make sure you communicate frequently. When patients send payments to you, immediately notify the collection agency. Try to avoid duplication of effort on the same account.

Annual audit and regular monitoring: Your relationship with your collection agency doesn't extend into perpetuity, so review it at least annually. Each month, review reports to make sure that the recovery rate meets your standards. If you are satisfied with the collection agency that you have chosen but are unhappy with a particular staff member, ask to have that individual replaced. Review accounts that were closed and returned to you as uncollectible. Check your patient complaints to see if there have been any problems. Finally, ask to listen in on calls made to your patients to make sure you are happy with the vendor's service.

How Can Information Technology Help You Manage Your Revenue Cycle Management Program?

Information technology (IT) can provide many benefits to your practice. Chapter 12 provides a comprehensive overview of the topic. Here are suggestions of ways in which IT can help you with your revenue cycle management program.

New patient registration prior to patient visits: By capturing demographic and insurance information on new patients prior to the patient visit, you can verify insurance eligibility ahead of time.

Electronic communication of new patient information: When new patients contact your office for an appointment, attach your new patient information package to an email. You can request demographic and insurance information and include your office policies for appointments, for telephone advice, and for payment.

Taking advantage of payer-specific IT applications: Most health plans have enhanced their websites to enable physicians to perform a variety of functions. Once you have a user name and password, you can file claims and receive electronic remittance advice. You can also obtain information on plan administrative requirements and network participation by other physicians. In some instances, you can check the reimbursement schedule for your practice.

Automatic transfer of accounts to your collection agency: If you are using an external collection agency, you can use your practice management system to automatically transfer out those accounts that meet your agreed upon criteria.

Use of a pre-collect letter and suspension of internal statement processing: Many practice management systems allow you to automatically generate a pre-collect letter and suspend internal statement processing.

Automatic statement processing: Most practice management systems automatically generate statements.

Pre-bill edits in your practice management system: Some newer practice management systems have built-in pre-bill edits that prompt you to correct claims before you submit them incorrectly. This feature immediately alerts your staff to problems that they can correct before the claim actually goes to the payer.

Writing down gross charges to net charges: Because most payers reimburse you at a level that is lower than your gross charges, leaving your gross charges on your books provides a false impression of the amount you can collect. Check to make sure that your practice management system writes your gross charges down to net charges. Your net charges are the more realistic representation of your accounts receivable.

Entering employer master and insurance master information: In some practice management systems, you can enter information that is specific to particular employers and payers so that you do not repeatedly have to enter the same information.

Where Can You Obtain Help If You Need It?

If you would like external help with your revenue cycle management program, consider talking with a general practice management consultant, a vendor to which you can outsource your entire billing and collection function, and/or a collection vendor with whom you share responsibility.

Good sources of additional information on revenue cycle management are:

▸ *Looking for the Cashcow. Action Steps to Improve Cash Flow in Medical Group Practices* by Thomas G. Hajny. (Edited by Kerstin B. Lynam, MGMA, 2000).

▸ *Operating Policies and Procedures Manual for Medical Practices*, 2nd Edition by Bette A. Warn and Elizabeth W. Woodcock. (MGMA, 2001).

▸ Articles available on-line from American Academy of Family Physicians (www.aafp. org/fpm):

  Aymond, R. (1999). Monitoring Your Practice's Financial Data: 10 Vital Signs.
  Capko, J. (1998). Questions to Ask About Your Accounts Receivable.
  Valancy, J. (1998). Finding Out How Much Your Plans Are Really Paying You.

References
1   Warn BA, Woodcock EW. *Operating Policies and Procedures Manual for Medical Practices*. (2e) Englewood, CO: MGMA; 2001.
2   Glass KP. *RVUs. Applications for Medical Practice Success*. Englewood, CO: MGMA; 2003.

Human Resources

The people who work with you and for you are your practice's most important assets. Regardless of the thought you put into organizing your practice, developing a strategic plan, creating a sound financial foundation, creating a marketing strategy, complying with federal and state laws and regulations, and purchasing information technology that supports your practice, the success of each of these aspects of practice management depends on the physicians with whom you practice and the administrative and clinical staff that support you.

This chapter was written with the assistance of Barnett Satinsky of Fox Rothschild LLP, Philadelphia, PA. It addresses the following questions:

- As an employer, what federal, state, and local laws affect your relationship with your employees?
- What recruitment strategies can you use to hire and retain good employees?
- What are the elements of an effective employee orientation program?
- What type of training should you provide for your employees?
- How should you develop a total compensation package that includes wages and benefits?
- How should you design your facilities to meet employee needs?
- What strategies can you use to encourage job stability?
- How should you address employee grievances?
- What are the features of a good performance evaluation system?
- How should you handle disciplinary action?
- How should you deal with employee resignations, terminations, and other departures from your practice?
- How can you deal with the diverse demographics of the twenty-first century workplace?
- What are good resources on employee human resource management?

As an Employer, What Federal, State, and Local Laws Affect Your Relationship with Your Employees?

Although you may identify yourself as a medical or surgical specialist, you also are a business owner. Make sure you understand your responsibilities as an employer. The federal, state, and local laws that dominate the human resource world of all industries affect you too. Just as you strive to remain well-informed in the clinical area in which you specialize, make sure you understand the legal environment in which you operate your business and employ your staff. Your attorney is the best source of information. This section provides general guidance.

Pay attention to four important areas, job discrimination, sexual and other types of harassment in the workplace, the Family and Medical Leave Act (FMLA), and the Americans with Disabilities Act (ADA). As suggested in the MGMA book *Tracking Hot HR Trends*,[1] you should be knowledgeable not only about the laws themselves, but also about emerging trends suggested by recent court cases.

Job discrimination can take many forms. Exhibit 7.1 lists the applicable federal laws, the groups they protect, and the relevant enforcement agencies (this exhibit can also be found on the website www.radcliffe-oxford.com/medicalpracticemanagement).

EXHIBIT 7.1 Laws that apply to job discrimination

LAW	GROUP PROTECTED	ENFORCEMENT AGENCY
Title VII of the Civil Rights Act of 1964 Civil Rights Act of 1991 Section 1981 of the Civil Rights Act of 1964	▸ Covers employment decisions based on race, gender, age (40 and older), religion, or national origin in businesses with 15 or more employees ▸ Places burden of proof on employer and permits compensatory and punitive monetary damages for discrimination	Equal Employment Opportunity Commission
Pregnancy Discrimination Act of 1978	▸ Amendment to Title VII that protects against discrimination based on pregnancy, childbirth, or related medical conditions in businesses with 15 or more employees ▸ Applies to hiring, terms and conditions of employment, health insurance, and fringe benefits	Equal Employment Opportunity Commission
Fair Labor Standards Act of 1938 and amendments	▸ Regulates wages, hours, records and reports, and child labor ▸ Applies to compensation for exempt and nonexempt employees ▸ Includes exemption tests	U.S. Department of Labor, Wage and Hour Division
Age Discrimination in Employment Act of 1987	▸ Protects people aged 40+ ▸ Applies to recruitment and employment by employers with 20 or more employees	Equal Employment Opportunity Commission
Family and Medical Leave Act of 1993 (FMLA)	▸ Applies to employers with 50 or more employees within 75 miles of the work site ▸ Allows employees 12 weeks' unpaid leave to care for a child after birth (or placement for adoption or foster care), to care for the serious health condition of a family member (e.g., child, spouse, parent), or for the employee if a serious health condition prohibits him/her from performing the job ▸ Gives employer the option to pay the employee for time away from the workplace ▸ Requires consistency in policy for all FMLA leaves	US Department of Labor, Wage and Hour Division

(continued)

LAW	GROUP PROTECTED	ENFORCEMENT AGENCY
Americans with Disabilities Act of 1990 (ADA)	▶ Applies to public and private employers with 15 or more employees ▶ Prohibits discrimination against people with physical or mental disabilities in employment, government programs and services, and public accommodation ▶ Applies to interviewing, hiring, the application process, testing, disciplinary actions, medical exams, compensation, job training, assignments, leave, layoffs, promotions, discharge and benefits. Covered employers must make "reasonable" accommodations for disabled people to perform the essential functions of a job ▶ In medical practices, also protects the right of patients not to be denied medical services because of their health conditions	Equal Employment Opportunity Commission

Sexual harassment is "unwelcome sexual advances, requests for sexual favors, and other verbal or physical conduct of a sexual nature" when:

▶ Submission to such conduct is made either explicitly or implicitly a term or condition of an individual's employment; or

▶ Submission to, or rejection of, such conduct by an individual is used as the basis for employment decisions affecting such individuals; or

▶ Such conduct has the purpose or effect of unreasonably interfering with an individual's work performance or creating an intimidating, hostile or offensive work environment.[1]

Court cases that have reached the US Supreme Court have established a new standard for employer liability for sexual harassment by supervisors and co-workers. Questions about sexual harassment of the same sex have also occurred as more gay and lesbian relationships become public and with the recognition that persons of either sex may be the aggressors. In some instances, state and local laws have been more protective against such discrimination than federal laws. Exhibit 7.2 suggests steps you can take to protect your employees against sexual harassment.

EXHIBIT 7.2 Steps you can take to protect your employees against sexual harassment in the workplace

▶ Hire carefully so you employ people who can do the job. Don't make sexual orientation a reason to hire or not hire a job candidate.

▶ Develop a formal policy against sexual harassment for your practice and post it where it is visible to everyone in the practice. Discuss the policy during employee and physician orientation and at staff meetings.

▶ Ask every employee to sign a written statement indicating that he/she understands your practice's sexual harassment policy.

▶ Include the sexual harassment policy in the employee handbook.

▶ Carefully train your supervisors to stop such conduct even if no complaint is filed.

▶ Apply your policies fairly and consistently.

If, despite your best efforts, one of your employees makes a complaint of sexual harassment in the workplace, immediately take action. Exhibit 7.3 suggests the steps you should take and can be found on the website www.radcliffe-oxford.com/medicalpracticemanagement.

Sexual harassment is not the only type of harassment that you should seek to avoid. Many federal courts have extended the protection of Title VII to the other protected categories mentioned in Exhibit 7.1: race, religion, national origin, and disability.

Taking a proactive approach applies to FMLA and ADA as well as to sexual harassment. Exhibits 7.4 and 7.5 offer suggestions to guide you and can be found on the website www.radcliffe-oxford.com/medicalpracticemanagement.

In addition to the laws mentioned above, be aware of other government regulations that affect your role as an employer. These are the Fair Credit Reporting Act, state Workers' Compensation laws, and the Occupational Safety and Health Act (OSHA).

What Recruitment Strategies Can You Use to Hire and Retain Good Employees?

Recruiting staff for your practice is a process, not a single activity. It involves clearly articulating your practice's mission, goals, and priorities, setting employee-specific goals, determining job requirements, creating a job description, advertising the position, reviewing applications, conducting interviews, making a decision, checking references, and extending a job offer. If you are careful in these steps, you can set a firm foundation for an ongoing performance evaluation program once the employee has been hired.

Step 1: Articulate Your Practice's Mission, Goals, Priorities, and Values

All medical practices are not created equal with respect to mission, goals, priorities, and values. If you are opening a new private practice, your short-term focus is on successful start-up. If you are an existing practice, you may be considering adding physicians, opening satellite offices, and making enhancements in your information technology. Regardless of your stage in the evolution of your practice, you'll have values that are important to you. Begin your recruitment process with a clear articulation of what you are and the direction in which you are going in the short term and the long term. Exhibit 7.6 contains an example for two pediatric practices. Their missions are similar, but their goals, priorities, and values differ.

EXHIBIT 7.6 Sample mission, goals, priorities, and values for two practices

	PEDIATRIC PRACTICE A	PEDIATRIC PRACTICE B
Mission	▸ Provide quality pediatric and adolescent care to the community	▸ Provide quality pediatric and adolescent care to the community
Goals	▸ Address the changing needs of a culturally diverse patient base	▸ Stabilize the practice's administrative and financial foundations
Priorities	▸ Replace the retiring practice manager ▸ Open a satellite office to better serve the western part of the county ▸ Select and implement EHR in the practice	▸ Replace the current office manager with an individual with more experience in financial management and human resources ▸ Recruit a full clinical team and concentrate on job stability

(*continued*)

	PEDIATRIC PRACTICE A	PEDIATRIC PRACTICE B
Important values	‣ Decision-making by physician consensus ‣ Open discussion ‣ Respect for the input of all members of the workforce	‣ More hands-on management by the three owners of the practice

Step 2: State the Position Goals

Once you have articulated the mission, goals, priorities, and values for your practice, identify the goals for the position for which you are hiring. For example, if you are Pediatric Practice A in Exhibit 7.6 and you are replacing your retiring practice manager, you'll want to consider candidates who can handle two big projects, opening a satellite office and introducing EHR into your practice. If you are Pediatric Practice B, however, the office manager whom you are recruiting will have different goals. Exhibit 7.7 contains a partial list of goals for Practice A's new practice manager.

EXHIBIT 7.7 Partial list of goals for practice manager

‣ Assess current practice workflow and identify strengths and weaknesses.

‣ Manage the process for selecting and implementing a vendor for EHR, including but not limited to describing practice needs, identifying potential vendors and products, developing Requests for Information, reviewing proposals, checking references, making site visits, selecting vendors, negotiating vendor contracts, and coordinating implementation.

‣ Plan and manage transition to new satellite office.

Step 3: State Job Requirements

Once you have stated the position goals, move on to job requirements. Does the job require special knowledge, skills, and abilities? Does it require completion of a certain number of years of education or special certification? Does it involve special physical capabilities (e.g., heavy lifting)?

If you are anxious to "just hire" and skip these early steps in the recruitment process, reconsider. The healthcare job market is volatile. People change jobs all the time for personal and economic reasons, and so the pool of applicants may be large. Make sure you understand your practice's needs and the characteristics of a job applicant who is most likely to carry out the goals you have listed. Exhibit 7.8 describes the experience of Turtle Bay Obstetrics & Gynecology, a four-physician practice in the Great Lakes region that made a hasty hiring decision that it came to regret.

EXHIBIT 7.8 Turtle Bay Obstetrics & Gynecology's mistake in hiring a new practice manager

Turtle Bay Obstetrics & Gynecology had four physicians. Following the departure of the practice manager, the billing supervisor expressed interest in the vacant position. The physicians were inexperienced in recruiting and were greatly relieved when an existing employee came forward. Without taking the time to identify the practice's mission, goals, priorities, and values or to list the position goals and requirements, the physicians made a job offer. Within three months, the practice was in a state of chaos. The new practice manager lacked the supervisory experience needed to manage a staff of 30. She had minimal knowledge of human resources, and employees claimed they were being treated unfairly. When employees who had been with the practice for many years threatened to leave, the physicians realized they had made a mistake. With the assistance of an external consultant, they developed the appropriate profile of their practice and a clear statement of job goals and requirements. They reorganized the practice, asked the practice manager to leave, and replaced her with a qualified candidate whom they recruited from outside the practice and who had previously managed a similar practice.

Step 4: Develop a Formal Job Description

Fourth, use your position goals and job requirements as the foundation for a formal job description that you can provide for individuals who are interested in the position. Exhibit 7.9, below, provides a recommended format for all job descriptions in your practice and Exhibit 7.10 provides a sample job description and can be found on the website www.radcliffe-oxford.com/medicalpracticemanagement. Another good resource is the questionnaire available on the website of the American Academy of Family Practice (http://aafp.org/fpm/20051000/jobdescription/pdf). As you review Exhibits 7.9 and 7.10, pay attention to the details. First, clarify the reporting relationship. Dual reporting relationships can be recipes for failure. Second, clarify the required levels of initiative and independence. For example, if you want a practice manager who follows the physicians' directions and is not expected to take initiative, recruit a follower, not a leader. Third, be clear about the scope of supervisory responsibility.

EXHIBIT 7.9 Recommended format for job descriptions

- ▶ Job title
- ▶ Reporting relationship
- ▶ Span of control/supervisory responsibilities
- ▶ Required initiative/leadership
- ▶ General summary of duties and responsibilities
- ▶ Priority and secondary functions
- ▶ Working conditions
- ▶ Physical and mental effort required
- ▶ Time commitment/indication of flexible hours
- ▶ Performance requirements:
  - — Knowledge, skills, and abilities
  - — Education
  - — Experience
  - — Certification
  - — Licenses
  - — Alternatives to minimum qualifications
- ▶ Leadership, decision-making, and initiative required.

Step 5: Spread the Word about Your Vacant Position

Once you have the job description, you can spread the word about your opportunity. If you are an existing practice and you encourage current employees to apply for vacant positions, post the job internally. If you decide to recruit outside your practice, take advantage of one or more free recruiting methods. Talk with medical colleagues and ask your employees if they know qualified people. State and regional chapters of the Medical Group Management Association of America (MGMA) meet regularly and often offer job search assistance to members and to practices that are recruiting new staff. If you have a practice website, you can post job opportunities there.

If the methods suggested above don't produce one or more qualified applicants, consider paid advertising. Remember that paid advertising can be expensive, so be thoughtful in your selection of newspapers or journals. Sometimes small town or neighborhood newspapers produce better results than large and more expensive daily papers. If you are doing a national search, use the MGMA recruiting service or a similar service offered by your professional specialty society's administrative organization. Make sure that whatever free and paid recruitment methods you use show your commitment to equal employment and ADA by producing an adequate pool of women, minorities, mature, and disabled workers.

Step 6: Review the Resumes that You Receive

After you have talked with colleagues and/or advertised the position, ask one individual in your practice to review the letters and resumes that you receive and divide them into two groups, qualified and not qualified for the position. As a courtesy to the applicants and as a method of reducing phone calls to your practice, notify all applicants that you have received the applications. When you eliminate candidates, let them know and thank them for their interest. Tell those applicants whom you are still considering your timetable for interviewing and making a decision.

Step 7: Conduct Telephone Interviews

Once you have narrowed the group of qualified applicants down to six to eight people, obtain additional information and a sense of the applicants' telephone skills through brief phone interviews. Then pare your list down even more and invite only the best candidates in for personal interviews.

Step 8: Conduct Personal Interviews

Preparation for personal interviews of qualified candidates is important. Develop a standard list of interview questions that you ask every applicant. Exhibit 7.11 contains suggested questions and can be found on the website www.radcliffe-oxford.com/medicalpracticemanagement. Be sure you understand the federal and state laws that govern the interview process. The language that you use is as important as the questions that you ask. Use the suggestions in Exhibit 7.12, which can be found on www.radcliffe-oxford.com/medicalpracticemanagement to help you phrase your questions in a way that doesn't violate any legal prohibitions.

By definition, working in a medical practice requires teamwork. Many practices ask prospective candidates to meet with other members of the practice. For example, if you are hiring a nurse, make sure to include administrative staff as well as clinical staff in the interview process.

Step 9: Contact References

After you have completed your interviews and asked other staff members to meet with the top candidates, narrow your selection to two or three people. At this point, with applicant permission, contact references and check credentials. Ask each reference the same set of questions. Exhibit 7.13 provides suggestions.

EXHIBIT 7.13 Suggested questions for references

> ▶ When did this individual work for your organization?
>
> ▶ What job did this individual perform?
>
> ▶ Did the individual carry out his/her responsibilities to your satisfaction? If not, why not?
>
> ▶ Did you encounter any problems with this individual's performance? If so, what were they?
>
> ▶ As a potential future employer, is there anything else I should know about this individual's ability to perform his/her job?

Step 10: Perform Criminal and Background Checks

As an employer in the medical field, you should be particularly careful about performing both criminal and background checks. The financial penalties and/or repercussions for billing fraud and clinical incompetence are severe. Two practical steps can help you accomplish this step easily. First, engage an outside service to do the criminal and background checks. Second, ask those employees who require professional certification or licensure to sign a statement indicating they will maintain these credentials.[2]

Step 11: Extend a Job Offer

When you are ready to extend a job offer to your top candidate, call the person on the phone, make the offer, and then follow up with a written offer letter. The offer letter is different from an employment contract, and for some employees you may want both. Include the title of the job, starting date, reporting relationship, job description, benefits and eligibility dates, and description of your probationary period (if you have one). If your offer is contingent on the results of pre-employment drug screening, make that requirement clear. Exhibit 7.14 contains a sample offer letter and can be found on the website www.radcliffe-oxford. com/medicalpracticemanagement. Exhibit 7.15 contains a sample list of employee benefits. Attach the benefit information to the offer letter so the individual to whom you are offering the job can consider this

EXHIBIT 7.15 Sample list of employee benefits

> ▶ Health insurance
>
> ▶ Dental insurance
>
> ▶ Short-term disability

- Long-term disability
- Life insurance
- Pension and profit sharing
- Tuition reimbursement
- Flex/Plan combining sick, vacation, and holiday

What Are the Elements of an Effective Employee Orientation Program?

When your new employee arrives at your practice, introduce him/her to the administrative and clinical members of your workforce, including physicians. If you have just filled a vacant position or if recruitment has taken a long time, you may be tempted to ask your new employee to begin right away. Providing orientation first is a better approach.

Give your practice manager, nurse manager, or other employee in a supervisory position clear responsibility for developing and implementing your orientation program. Exhibit 7.16 provides a suggested list of topics to be included.

EXHIBIT 7.16 Suggested topics for employee orientation

- History of your practice
- Mission, goals, priorities
- Values
- Benefit options
- Organization chart
- Responsibilities of administrative and clinical personnel
- Methods of communication (e.g., telephone, email, written, meetings)
- Guidelines for customer service
- Code of conduct
- Confidentiality
- Important laws: HIPAA, OSHA, FMLA, ADA
- Job description
- Employee relations
- Training

Make orientation a job requirement, not an option, and make sure you compensate employees for their time.

People learn in different ways, so reinforce your message by using different teaching methods. For example, you can ask new employees to watch a short video about your practice and give them a copy to watch at home. Take them on a tour of your entire facility, including satellite locations. Give them an employee handbook that they can read at their leisure. Exhibit 7.17 contains topics that the manual should include and can be found on the website www.radcliffe-oxford.com/medicalpracticemanagement.

Request employee feedback on your orientation program and make changes based on the suggestions that you receive.

Orientation is important not only for new employees, but also for current employees. At least once each year meet with your entire workforce and re-orient them to the important aspects of your practice.

What Type of Training Should You Provide for Your Employees?

Both the administrative and clinical aspects of healthcare change regularly. As an employer, make sure that your employees remain certified in their particular areas of expertise and up-to-date on new developments.

Clinical and technical staff will be required to obtain continuing education units (CEUs) to maintain their certification. Provide financial support and opportunities for employees to attend relevant training sessions. Include the cost of employee training in your budget so you are not put in the position of responding to individual requests.

Encourage the employees who are involved in managing your practice to participate in MGMA national, state, and regional education programs and in managers' groups organized by your particular specialty. All of these groups offer excellent information and networking opportunities.

In addition to supporting professional training for your employees, promote their professional growth and development by holding regular staff meetings and by making sure that managers and supervisors meet regularly with individual employees. Use your staff meetings to share information, build teamwork, and jointly solve problems. Meetings with individual employees help employees and supervisors ensure that work is performed in the desired way and that goals are achieved. Spare your employees any surprises at their annual performance evaluations by providing ongoing guidance and feedback.

How Should You Develop a Total Compensation Package that Includes Salary/Wages and Benefits?

As an employer, you are offering your employees a total compensation package that includes both salary/wages and benefits. In many practices, the benefits may represent as much as 30 percent of the wages. The Fair Labor Standards Act (FLSA) governs the minimum hourly wage and payment for overtime and on-call hours.

With respect to wage and salary levels, you can use a variety of methods to determine how you will pay your employees. Exhibit 7.18 provides four suggestions.[3]

EXHIBIT 7.18 Methods for determining wage and salary levels

METHOD	COMMENT
Point methods	Assign points to compensable factors that are identified in each job. Add up the points and translate them into dollars. This approach is similar to using Relative Value Units in clinical work.
Job classification systems	Classify jobs based on job content and job requirements. Then put them into job categories with assigned pay ranges.
Wage and salary surveys	Use market information available from MGMA and other professional organizations as benchmarks for your practice.
Combination of methods	Recognize both objective job factors and the labor market in determining wage and salary levels.

Once you have a formal wage and salary scale, address the following related issues:[1] annual cost-of-living and/or merit increases and reward and recognition programs.[3] Some practices give all employees an across the board cost-of-living increase regardless of performance. Other practices offer a merit increase based on performance or some combination of cost-of-living and merit pay. With respect to special reward and recognition programs, employees appreciate employee-of-the-month programs, personal thank-you notes, designated parking spaces, and other symbols of thanks.

Regardless of how you set and upgrade your wage and salary scale, communicate your methodology to your employees. Perceived inequity in compensation can be a major source of tension in the workplace. If you have a system, let people know what it is and how you apply it fairly to everyone in your practice.

Regardless of the way in which you determine your wage and salary scale, keep payroll information confidential and locked in a secure place.

With respect to benefits, you have choices in what you offer and in your packaging. Exhibit 7.19 lists the employee benefits that many practices offer, as well as some of your options (this exhibit can also be found on the website www.radcliffe-oxford.com/medicalpracticemanagement).

EXHIBIT 7.19 Sample employee benefits

EMPLOYEE BENEFIT	CONSIDERATIONS
Health insurance	▶ You can make coverage effective upon employment or after a specified time period (e.g., 30 days after start date). ▶ You can cover or not cover employee spouses and dependents. ▶ You can offer a Health Savings Account (HSA).
Dental insurance	▶ You can make this effective upon employment or after a specified time period (e.g., 30 days after start date). ▶ You can cover or not cover employee spouses and dependents. ▶ You can decide not to offer this benefit at all.
Long- and short-term disability insurance	
Life insurance	
Retirement plan	
Time off for holidays, sick, vacation days	▶ You can offer this as a single paid time off (PTO) package or as separate benefits. ▶ You can link the time off to longevity with your practice.
Other leave time: disability, military, jury duty, bereavement, inclement weather	▶ You are not required to pay for any leave time. ▶ With respect to disability, treat childbirth like any other disability. ▶ You cannot penalize employees for serving military or jury duty, even though you are not required to pay for this time out of the office. ▶ Some leave requirements are governed by federal and state law (military) and some by state law (jury duty).
Education/tuition assistance	▶ If you offer this benefit, specify requirements.
Parking	
Other	

How Should You Design Your Facilities to Meet Employee Needs?

As an employer, it is your responsibility to make the workplace environment safe and comfortable for your employees. The Occupational Safety and Health Administration (OSHA) names ten controls to prevent and mitigate the effects of workplace hazards, including violence by patients and members of your workforce. Exhibit 7.20 lists these recommendations. Employees pay a lot of attention to the environment in which they work, so don't stop with OSHA. Take additional steps to meet common employee needs. Exhibit 7.21 provides suggestions.

EXHIBIT 7.20 OSHA-recommended controls to prevent workplace hazards

▶ Alarm systems and panic buttons

▶ Convex mirrors, elevated vantage points, clear visibility of service and cash register areas

▶ Bright interior and exterior lighting

▶ Adequate staffing

▶ Arrangement of furniture to prevent entrapment

▶ Physical barriers such as pass-through windows or deep service counters

▶ Emergency procedures in case of robbery

▶ Training to identify hazardous situations and appropriate responses

▶ Video surveillance equipment and closed-circuit TV

▶ Availability of stress reduction programs and counseling for employees

EXHIBIT 7.21 Suggested features of your facility that address common employee needs

FEATURE	SUGGESTION
Parking	▶ Provide free parking for employees.
Storage of personal items	▶ Provide lockers where employees can store their personal belongings.
Employee lounge and kitchen	▶ Allocate space where employees can take a break, eat lunch or dinner, etc. ▶ Equip it with a refrigerator, microwave, and table and chairs. ▶ Provide paper plates and utensils. ▶ Offer food and beverages from vending machines. ▶ Hang a bulletin board where you can post required government notices (e.g., compliance with ADA, FMLA, Civil Rights Act, HIPAA Notice of Privacy Practices). ▶ Provide a box for employee suggestions.
Restrooms	▶ Provide restrooms that are for employee use only.
Employee lounge	▶ Provide a private area where employees who are not feeling well can rest.
Library	▶ Provide a library or resource area.
Outside area	▶ Provide picnic tables and chairs.
Other	▶ Provide access to an exercise area, day care, etc.

What Strategies Can You Use to Encourage Job Stability?

Once you recruit, train, and motivate your employees to build an effective team for your practice, your goal should be employee retention. Several strategies can help you stabilize your work force. First, take human resource management seriously, and put policies and procedures in place as soon as possible. Communicate clearly with your employees rather than waiting for them to come to you with problems. Monitor your budget carefully. If you anticipate a decrease or fluctuation in patient revenue, consider using part-time and temporary staff and/or outside consultants so you can reduce the number of full-time employees that you have to pay.

Take time to get to know your employees. Greet them when you come into the office. Ask about their families without prying. Thank them for a good job. Although it may seem unimportant to you, schedule several social occasions during the year as a way of expressing your gratitude for their hard work.

Just as you take the pulse of your patients, take the pulse of your employees. Employee satisfaction surveys, frequent staff meetings, and regular meetings between supervisors and their employees are good ways to get employee feedback.

How Should You Address Employee Grievances?

A grievance procedure gives employees the opportunity to make complaints about issues in the workplace other than harassment. Just knowing that they have a formal way of complaining about management decisions tells employees that you respect their opinions, even if they differ from yours. Exhibit 7.22 provides suggestions for developing a grievance process for your practice.

EXHIBIT 7.22 Developing a grievance process for your practice

- Develop a clear and effective written grievance policy. You can restrict the policy to disagreements regarding the interpretation and application of company policies, rules, and handbooks, or make it broader.

- Include multiple review steps: by the immediate supervisor, by the supervisor's manager, and by senior management. A fourth review step, binding arbitration by an outside arbitrator, is optional. Some employers don't like outside arbitration because the provision forces them to give up their own rights to making final decisions in the workplace.

- If you already have a grievance policy for your practice, review the language. Make sure the policy clearly states the requirement that employees follow the policy even if they disagree with management's actions.

- Review your grievance policy with legal counsel.

- Communicate the policy to your employees in several ways. Include it in your employee handbook. Mention it during orientation, and remind employees about the policy during training that you provide on a regular basis.

What Are the Features of a Good Performance Evaluation Program?

One of the most effective ways to relate each employee's individual goals to his/her actual performance is to develop a formal performance evaluation program. Your system should have four goals, as described below.

‣ Provide a method for each employee and supervisor to collaborate in carrying out a historical evaluation of performance and setting of future goals.

‣ Incorporate into a single evaluation three important components: technical proficiencies that are customized for each role, organizational goals, and behavioral standards. The organizational goals and behavioral standards apply to everyone in your practice.

‣ Clearly describe, for each position, fully acceptable performance, exceptional performance, and performance that falls below standard.

‣ Provide a forum for employees and supervisors to exchange ideas on the employee's professional development for the coming year, ways in which the supervisor can enhance growth and development, and other resources and/or support that can contribute toward achievement of desired outcomes.

If you have been careful in your recruitment process, you already have a job description for each employee. Use it as the basis for a job checklist that identifies Goals/Functions and Technical Competencies for the position.

Once the employee and supervisor agree on both the job description and job checklist, use both to regularly review the employee's progress. For example, if the first few months of employment are considered a probationary period in your practice, do an evaluation at the end of that period. Do another evaluation mid-way during the year and do another one at the end of the year when you consider wage and salary increases and bonuses. Use the same instrument each time.

Since healthcare requires finely tuned teamwork, some employers incorporate a peer evaluation instrument into their performance evaluation systems. The employee asks the supervisor and peers of his/her choosing to provide feedback directly to the supervisor. The supervisor then combines the information into a single comprehensive document.

Appendix F contains a complete performance evaluation program, including a peer evaluation instrument, sample job checklists and job-specific competencies and expectations, a sheet for setting future goals, suggested questions for the supervisor, a method for scoring performance evaluations, and a cover sheet. Appendix F can be found on the website www.radcliffe-oxford.com/medicalpracticemanagement. Another good resource is the American College of Physicians website. See www.acponline.org/private/pmc/effprsnl.pdf.

How Should You Handle Disciplinary Action?

All employers encounter situations that warrant disciplinary action against employees. In spite of your best efforts to collaborate with your employees in setting and achieving goals, some people won't achieve the desired level of competence. Others will deliberately or inadvertently break important rules that your practice has established, documented, and communicated to your entire workforce. If you are smart, you'll develop an approach to disciplinary action shortly after you set your practice up, rather than when you need it in a hurry.

Aspen Publishing's *Medical Group Practice: Legal and Administrative Guide*[2] provides practical suggestions for dealing with both discipline and discharge. Exhibit 7.23 contains a condensed version of this information and can also be found on the website www.radcliffe-oxford.com/medicalpracticemanagement.

EXHIBIT 7.23 Suggestions for disciplinary action and discharge

Things you should do:

▶ Develop and maintain specific written work rules.

▶ Communicate your work rules to your employees in an employee manual, posted work rules, and/or regular meetings.

▶ Document minor and major violations.

▶ Develop a system for progressive disciplinary action that you apply consistently except in the case of certain serious violations. For example, if you discovered that one of your employees had embezzled money, you would fire the employee immediately.

▶ Keep a log of all disciplinary action that you administer. Make sure that one person in your practice maintains this record.

▶ Before taking disciplinary action, contact the person who maintains the log to make sure that disciplinary action in your practice is consistent.

▶ Discipline an employee when the violation first occurs or as soon as you have completed your investigation.

▶ Investigate the circumstances thoroughly by interviewing participants and witnesses and by taking written statements.

▶ If a union is involved and an employee requests that a union representative attend an investigative interview, allow the employee the opportunity to have a union steward present.

▶ If no union is involved and an employee requests a co-worker be allowed to attend an investigative interview, allow the employee the opportunity to have a co-worker present as a witness and advisor to the employee, but not as a direct participant.

▶ Inform the employee that the goal of disciplinary action (other than discharge) is correction, not punishment.

▶ Do progressive employee disciplining for the same or similar conduct.

▶ Maintain all disciplinary write-ups for at least two years.

▶ When writing disciplinary action, incorporate prior action(s) taken.

▶ When writing disciplinary action, notify the employee of likely action if there are future violations.

Things you should not do:

▶ Don't give oral discipline without documenting your action and placing the information in the appropriate file.

▶ Don't file disciplinary action slips without first obtaining the signature(s) of the employee or a witness to the discipline.

▶ Don't apply different disciplinary actions for the same or similar conduct by different employees without a valid reason.

▶ Don't discipline or discharge an employee without a thorough investigation.

▶ Don't discipline or discharge an employee without thorough documentation.

▶ Don't discipline or discharge an employee without first allowing the person being disciplined or discharged the opportunity to explain his/her position.

▶ Don't discipline or discharge an employee for violation of a rule that the employer failed to communicate or which any employee is deemed to know (e.g., don't embezzle money).

▶ Don't take into consideration age, gender, or race when determining discipline or discharge.

▶ Don't rely on your memory to remember employee violations. Document them.

How Should You Deal with Employee Resignations, Discharges, and Other Departures from your Practice?

Regard employee resignations, discharges, and other departures from your practice as a part of doing business. Regardless of how careful you have been during the hiring process and how much thought you have given to job descriptions, developing and implementing a performance evaluation system, and providing regular feedback, people leave. Make sure you have clear a policy and procedures before you need them.

As your attorney will advise you, protect yourself against legal action for wrongful discharge. The legal concept of employment-at-will gives both the employer and the employee the right to end the relationship at any time for any reason. The concept does not, however, give you as the employer the right to discharge an employee for an unlawful reason such as age, race, or gender. Employees may also claim that the employment relationship was "permanent" or in some way guaranteed. Exhibit 7.24 suggests steps you can take to protect yourself against these and other legal actions and can also be found on the website www.radcliffe-oxford.com/medicalpracticemanagement.

EXHIBIT 7.24 Suggestions for avoiding problems related to employee departures from your practice

Resignations
▶ If an employee that you would like to keep resigns from your practice, make sure you understand the real as opposed to the stated reason. Talk with others in your practice about whether or not you can accommodate the employee's requests in an appropriate way. Agreeing to pay a higher salary is not necessarily a good response.

Discharges
▶ Check with legal counsel first, not afterwards.

▶ To protect your practice against the claim that the employment relationship was "permanent", include disclaimer language in your employee handbook. Suggested language is: "I understand that this policy handbook does not create a contract of employment and that as such, I may resign at any time I desire and the company may terminate my employment at any time, with or without notice, and for any reason."

▶ Avoid sudden firings. Document your complaints about the employee's performance using the multi-step process that you have in your practice. Give the employee every opportunity to improve before you take action.

▶ Make sure you understand the supervisor or manager's real reason for recommending discharge. Did the manager or supervisor violate a policy or procedure, make an arbitrary or capricious decision, discriminate in violation of federal and/or state laws or public policy, retaliate against the employee because of refusal to perform an illegal act, or interfere with an employee's constitutional right?

❱ With direction and feedback from legal counsel, prepare a letter that addresses the effective date, final pay (including any sick or vacation time that you owe the employee), severance pay (if any), vested pension rights, and employee benefits. Explain how the Consolidated Omnibus Budget Reconciliation Act (COBRA) works so the employee understands what will happen with health and dental benefits. You may ask the employee to sign a written waiver of claims in return for additional compensation.

❱ Plan ahead with respect to what you will say during the meeting, how you will handle references, and what you will tell the rest of your workforce.

❱ Provide the employee with a list of property that must be returned to you. Examples are keys, computers, and supplies.

❱ Ask a second person to accompany you to the meeting as a witness.

❱ Pick an appropriate time for the meeting. For example, the end of the week or the end of the day is preferable to Monday morning.

❱ Give the employee the opportunity to express his/her feelings.

State laws give employees the opportunity to file for Unemployment Compensation in certain circumstances. If an employee files a claim against your practice, check with legal counsel before you respond. Particularly in situations where you expect the employee to file another claim (e.g., discrimination), your response to the unemployment claim may have broader repercussions.

How Can You Deal with the Diverse Demographics of the Twenty-first Century Workplace?

The demographic characteristics of both the work force and the patient population in the twenty-first century are very different from what they were just a decade ago. The percentages of people of color, of people who have emigrated from foreign countries, and of people who are 65 and older have increased. According to the US Bureau of the Census, by 2020, more than 30 percent of the population will be culturally diverse. By 2080, what we call minorities today may represent more than 50 percent of the US population.[1]

An important implication of cultural diversity is religious diversity. Census figures count 1500 religious organizations, and the number is growing. The Equal Employment Opportunity Commission has received many legal claims based on employers' refusal to allow employees to freely express their religious beliefs.

You may already be familiar with the language that describes differences among generations.

❱ The GI Generation was born between 1901 and 1925. Now in the final decades of their lives, members of this group came of age with a strong sense of patriotism, family, and work. Many are still active and healthy, and they want to collaborate with their caregivers to stay that way. Their needs require more attention to geriatric care.

❱ The Silent Generation was born between 1926 and 1945. Many in this group are active seniors. They work, travel, and volunteer. Managed care insurance, with its emphasis on preventive care, became widespread during this group's prime working years, and many have continued that coverage into senior plans. This generation, like the one that preceded it, values hard work. When these people retire from the workforce, medical practices will feel a loss.

▶ Baby Boomers were born between 1945 and 1964. This group has been more inclined to explore alternatives to traditional occupations and careers. Boomers fought in and protested against the Vietnam War and engaged in civil rights activities. The group is large. Members tend to be "loners" rather than joiners. Baby Boomers don't like the idea of ageing, and they often turn to alternative medicine as a way to ward off old age. As employees, they may be interested in phased retirement plans.

▶ Generation X was born between 1965 and 1981. This group is smaller than the Baby Boomer group before it. Members are less supportive of institutional values and tend to create their own "virtual families" from their professional and personal lives. They are the primary users of obstetrics/gynecology, pediatric, and family practice care. Members of Generation X are smart consumers who are responsive to a variety of marketing techniques, particularly the Internet. When Generation X people are patients, there may be miscommunication between them and members of the Silent Generation. When this generation becomes healthcare providers themselves, there are many women among them who are striving for a healthy balance between career and family.

▶ Generation Y was born between 1982 and 2003. This generation is computer fluent. As employees, they will expect to apply for jobs electronically, and as employees, they will expect information technology to play an important role in their workplace environments.

Given the characteristics of cultural diversity and multiple generations in the workplace and patient populations, your role as an employer and caregiver can embrace or reject the reality. If you are willing to accept the changing demographics, you can be proactive in your strategies. Exhibits 7.25 and 7.26 provide suggestions.

EXHIBIT 7.25 Strategies for accommodating cultural and religious diversity in your workforce and patient population

---

▶ Promote and support attitudes, behaviors, knowledge, and skills necessary for staff to work together and provide patient care with respect for cultural diversity.

▶ Develop a management strategy that addresses cultural diversity in your practice. Establish goals, plans, policies, procedures, and identify responsible staff members.

▶ Solicit community and patient involvement in the development and implementation of patient care that recognizes cultural diversity.

▶ Develop and implement a strategy to recruit, retain, and promote qualified diverse and culturally competent clinical and support staff who can address the needs of the communities that you serve.

▶ Support ongoing education and training that addresses cultural diversity for all members of your workforce. For example, if many of your patients are Hispanic, help your employees obtain the required linguistic skills.

▶ Translate signage and patient information into one or more appropriate languages so that all patients can understand it.

▶ If needed, make sure that interpreters and bilingual staff can provide assistance to patients who need help.

▶ When you collect patient demographic information, make sure to record the primary spoken language.

▶ On an ongoing basis, obtain information about the changing demographics in your community and use it to guide your practice in the way in which you deliver healthcare services.

▶ Obtain information about the healthcare needs of populations in the community for which you provide care.

▶ Ensure that cultural diversity is formally integrated into your practice by incorporating it into your strategic business plan and the personal goals and objectives of all members of your workforce.

▶ Develop systems to develop complaints about cultural insensitivity.

▶ Prepare an annual report on the way in which you are addressing cultural diversity in the workforce and in your patient population.

Source: *Tracking Hot HR Trends.*[1]

EXHIBIT 7.26 Strategies for accommodating generational differences in your workforce and patient population

▶ Engage your management team in understanding and meeting the needs, attitudes, and preferences of each generation.

▶ Avoid stereotyping people in the different generational groups.

▶ If your practice provides care to patients of multiple generations, sensitize your clinicians to differences.

▶ Adjust your recruitment and retention strategies to meet the needs of different generations. Regardless of your strategies, be mindful of the appropriate legal context.

▶ Identify inter-generational problems in your workforce and between your workforce and patients so you can find creative solutions.

What Are Good Resources on Human Resource Management?

If you would like to learn more about human resource management in your practice, the references listed below contain helpful information.

▶ Aspen Reference Group Aspen Health Law Center. Medical Group Practice: *Legal and Administrative Guide*. Gaithersburg, MD: Aspen Publishers; 1999–2003.

▶ Dressler G. *A Framework for Human Resource Management*. Fourth Edition. Upper Saddle River, NJ: Pearson Prentice Hall; 2006.

▶ Fried BJ, Thomas MS, Goodrich LL. Human Resource Management. In: Keagy BA, Thomas MS, editors. *Essentials of Physician Practice Management*. San Francisco, CA: John Wiley & Sons, Inc.; 2004.

▶ Novak A, Price C. *Tracking Hot HR Trends*. Englewood, CO: Medical Group Management Association; 2001.

▸ Schryver DL, editor. An Assessment Manual for Medical Groups. Englewood, CO: Medical Group Management Association; 2002.

References

1   Novak A, Price C. *Tracking Hot HR Trends*. Englewood, CO: Medical Group Management Association; 2001.
2   Fried BJ, Thomas MS, Goodrich LL. Human Resource Management. In: Keagy BA, Thomas MS, editors. *Essentials of Physician Practice Management*. San Francisco, CA: John Wiley & Sons, Inc.; 2004.
3   Aspen Reference Group Aspen Health Law Center. *Medical Group Practice: Legal and Administrative Guide*. Gaithersburg, MD: Aspen Publishers; 1999–2003.

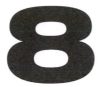

Physician Issues

This chapter addresses the following questions:

- How should you recruit new physicians into your practice?
- What steps can you take to retain physicians in your practice?
- What should you include in your physician orientation program?
- How should you develop a physician compensation plan?
- How can you develop a system for evaluating physician performance?
- How should you handle physician departures from your practice?
- Where can you learn more about the physician issues addressed in this chapter?

How Should You Recruit New Physicians into Your Practice?

Physician recruitment is a multi-step process that begins with a financial determination of whether or not your practice can afford to add an additional physician or replace a physician who has left your practice. Your goal should be to meet your practice's clinical needs and remain within your budget. It is not to bring into your practice every physician who expresses interest in joining you. In some cases, a non-physician provider such as a nurse practitioner or physician assistant may be more suitable than a physician.

Exhibit 8.1 describes a solo otolaryngology practice that hired a new part-time physician without first doing its financial homework. The outcome was a disaster.

EXHIBIT 8.1 Swan River Ear, Nose, & Throat's disastrous recruitment of a new physician

Dr Marcella and his wife, an audiologist, opened Swan River Ear, Nose, & Throat in 2002. By 2005, the practice was thriving, and the Marcellas decided that an additional part-time physician might contribute to the growth of the practice and enable Dr Marcella to share on-call hours with a colleague. Without doing a financial analysis, Dr Marcella contacted Dr Nare, an Air Force colleague whom he had met several years ago. Dr Nare and his family were anxious to relocate and they quickly purchased a new home in anticipation of the change. Without any formalities, Dr Marcella offered Dr Nare a part-time position. At no time during the interview process did the two physicians discuss Dr Marcella's expectations for productivity and interpersonal relations or Dr Nare's needs for space and support. When Dr Nare arrived on his first day at work, he expressed his desire for two offices and 1.5 additional FTEs. Dr Marcella acquiesced to Dr. Nare's request without determining the impact on the practice's bottom line. Within just three months,

Dr Marcella realized that he had made an inappropriate choice of a new physician and that he was now saddled with the cost of additional space and staff. Had Dr. Marcella taken the time to do a financial analysis in the first place, the outcome might have been different.

If, and only if, it makes good financial sense to recruit an additional physician, initiate your search. Your options are word of mouth, referrals from colleagues, contacts with academic medical centers, especially where you did your own training, national searches through advertising, and working with a professional physician recruitment firm. If you work with a recruitment firm, you can arrange either a contingency or a retained search. Exhibit 8.2 describes both approaches. The cost of working with a recruitment firm can range between 20 and 30 percent of the physician's salary for the first year.

EXHIBIT 8.2 Options in working with a professional physician recruitment firm

Contingency search	▸ Firm collaborates with an employer to fill a position.
	▸ Employer can often pursue its own search simultaneously.
	▸ Firm receives payment only if the employer hires a candidate that it presents.
	▸ Employer is not obligated to hire a candidate presented by the firm.
Retained search	▸ Firm collaborates with the employer on exclusive basis.
	▸ Employer and firm have a formal contract.
	▸ Firm works with the employer until the completion of search.
	▸ Employer generally pays fees at the outset and conclusion of the process.

Regardless of your approach to physician recruitment, allow six to nine months lead time. Candidates will want to meet with you and familiarize themselves with the community in which your practice is located. If both of you have preliminary interest, the candidate's family will want to make a follow-up visit. Family issues such as job opportunities for spouses and educational opportunities for children will become part of the equation. If you are recruiting a candidate from out of town, make sure you budget enough money to pay for travel expenses, entertainment, and relocation.

Keep in mind two potential barriers to recruitment, the location of your practice and your attitude toward information technology (IT). You can't do much about your location, but you can make sure that your approach to IT support is forward- not backward-looking. Chapter 7 on Human Resources describes generational differences in the workplace. Physicians who have recently completed their training are likely to prefer working in practices that use information technology, particularly electronic health records (EHR), to support practice operations.

One of the most challenging aspects of physician recruitment is going beyond the basic requirements of training and experience. Given your mission, goals, priorities, and values, will the candidate fit into your practice? And conversely, will you meet the candidate's requirements? Exhibit 8.3 suggests questions that you can ask physicians who are interested in joining a primary care practice, this exhibit can also be found on the website www.radcliffe-oxford.com/medicalpracticemanagement. Modify the questions to suit your specialty. Exhibit 8.4 identifies the typical concerns of a physician who is seeking a suitable practice opportunity.

EXHIBIT 8.3 Questions to ask physicians who want to join your practice

- Why do you want to join our practice?

- What are your short- and long-term goals?

- In our primary care practice, we expect full-time physicians to see 25 patients per day. Will you be comfortable with this expectation?

- We have designated one physician as our Managing Partner, and we ask other partners to assume the responsibility for particular projects under the Managing Partner's direction. Are you willing to assume administrative responsibility for one or more projects that interest you?

- We pride ourselves on our participation in committee activities of the two hospitals to which we admit patients. Will you be willing to represent us as needed?

- In our practice, we bring in new physicians as salaried employees for X number of years. Based on our assessment of clinical performance and ability to fit into our practice, we may eventually offer the opportunity for partnership. Are you comfortable with our approach or do you have different expectations?

- Teamwork is very important in our practice. Our entire clinical and administrative staff meets weekly to share information and identify and resolve problems. Does our philosophy of practice management correspond to your own?

- Identify some of the positive and negative attributes of your prior clinical setting. What specific things seemed to work well or not well in your previous practice setting?

- What do you consider to be the most frustrating aspect(s) of practicing medicine and how have you learned to cope with it (them)?

- Describe an ideal work day.

EXHIBIT 8.4 Typical concerns of a physician who is seeking a suitable practice opportunity

Location	• Geography: proximity to family, weather, educational opportunities. • Environment: urban, suburban, rural, population density and projections, convenience of basic family services like shopping, schools, convenience of services for patients.
Community	• Economy: cost of living compared to current place of residence, home, per capita income, potential to live close to practice (if desired). • Family interests: availability of work for spouse/significant other, social opportunities, leisure activities, employer attitude toward family commitments. • Children: public and private schools, special needs, organized activities, recreation, day care options and affordability. • Social interests: proximity to family and friends, restaurants, cultural activities, hobbies. • Religion: access to preferred denomination, cultural diversity, events. • Recreation: availability and accessibility of sports and hobbies.
Your practice	• Practice viability: size, stability, historical and projected volume, strategic business plan, marketing plan, financial history, managed care environment, clinical and administrative support, space, use of information technology (IT) to support practice operations, level of supervision, quality initiatives.

(continued)

Your practice (cont.)	▶ Research (optional): availability of seed money, research time, access to clinical lab, availability of opportunities for collaboration, track record of obtaining grants, administrative support, space, access to patients, equipment, credentialing, availability of state-of-the-art information systems. ▶ Teaching (optional): residents, fellows, medical students, academic appointment, tenure, career advancement, faculty practice plan, mentoring. ▶ Fiscal viability of practice: potential for growth, current and projected demand for service, payer mix, volume of visits/week, referral base or specialty network, current status of billing/collections, affiliations with colleagues, expected market changes, competition, use of physician extenders. ▶ Practice management: physician role in practice management, practice administrator/manager/office manager, billing/collection, coding, record keeping, managed care contracting, IT support, patient flow. ▶ Benefits: health and dental insurance, long- and short-term disability insurance, pension and profit sharing, parking, administrative support. ▶ Salary and other financial information: method of physician compensation, opportunity for paid administrative opportunities, salary range, potential for bonus, allocation of overhead costs, relocation allowance, sign-on bonus, income guarantee, paid malpractice premiums, free office space, loan forgiveness programs. ▶ Parameters for equity buy-in.

Adopted from "How to Find the Perfect Job" by Jill Berger-Fiffy[1].

After you and your partners meet with several candidates, make your decision and draft both an offer letter and a written contract that will be a binding employment agreement. Exhibit 8.5 contains a sample offer letter of employment, and Exhibit 8.6 identifies topics that should be included in the written physician employment contract, both of these exhibits can be found on the website, www.radcliffe-oxford.com/medicalpracticemanagement. If your new physician is an independent contractor as opposed to an employee, some of the topics in Exhibit 8.6 will differ.

What Steps Can You Take to Retain Physicians in Your Practice?

Physician recruiting is time-consuming and expensive, so once you find someone suitable for your practice, make sure you take appropriate steps to encourage physician retention. By anticipating and meeting common physician needs, you can increase practice stability and minimize unwanted physician turnover.

The rule of thumb here is "Plan Ahead." Provide excellent clinical working conditions, including but not limited to adequate space, qualified clinical and administrative support, and clear communication. With respect to specific equipment, respond to requests from individual physicians by looking at the value to the entire practice. Start with the services that you want to offer, and then discuss equipment. If the service makes financial sense and the new equipment will help you develop that service, make the purchase. Include both the service and the equipment in your operating and capital budgets.

As the business of medicine becomes more challenging, more physicians are assuming managerial roles in their practices by becoming the Managing Partners. Make sure you compensate and motivate your colleagues who are willing to take on administrative duties. Without them, you wouldn't have a practice.

Finally, schedule social events to welcome new physicians into your practice and to help them and their families make a smooth adjustment. Relocation is one of life's more difficult challenges.

What Should You Include in Your Physician Orientation Program?

When a new physician joins your practice as a partner or as a salaried or contracted employee, require that he/she participate in a formal physician orientation program. Every medical practice is unique, and you want to be sure that new physicians understand how you manage your practice, your expectations of physicians, and the ways in which your values and culture affect daily operations. For legal reasons, provide comprehensive guidance including written material. Don't assume that new physicians will "just know" what to do or "pick up information as they go along."

A formal physician orientation program should address at least the topics listed in Exhibit 8.7.

EXHIBIT 8.7 Contents of physician orientation program

- History of your practice
- Mission, goals, priorities, values
- Practice patterns: hospital privileges, use of outside lab and other ancillary services
- Image that you strive to project in your community
- Financial history of your practice
- Participation in managed care networks and public programs (e.g., Medicare, Medicaid, etc.)
- Administrative and clinical organization
- Strategic plan
- Marketing plan
- Disaster plan
- Risk management
- Quality assurance
- Process for becoming a partner in your practice
- Physician expectations: productivity, practice development and growth, leadership
- Performance evaluations
- Billing and coding
- Compliance with applicable laws and regulations: Stark, Anti-Kickback, OSHA, HIPAA Privacy and Security, FMLA, ADA, etc.

In addition to providing formal orientation to new physicians, consider assigning one of your current physicians as a mentor to your new recruit. The mentor can facilitate your new physician's development both inside and outside of your practice. Particularly when a new physician has little past clinical experience, the mentor can provide guidance. The mentor can also help foster the practice's specific culture and values in new physicians. Outside the practice, the mentor can introduce the new physician to medical colleagues and to the hospital(s) to which you admit patients.

How Should You Develop a Physician Compensation Plan?

Physician compensation is a sensitive subject. By establishing a formal process for reviewing your compensation plan, you can minimize dissension among your partners. An eleven-step process is described below.

▶ First, identify a compensation committee so the process is participative. Ask multiple physicians within your practice to form a Compensation Redesign Task Force. Their early involvement will enhance the willingness of all the partners to reach consensus. Also, decide how you will involve your practice manager. Some practices ask the practice manager to direct the process, obtain information, and compare alternatives. Using the information that has been organized for them, the physicians make the ultimate decision.

▶ Second, make sure you understand relevant legal issues.

▶ Third, determine your goals.

▶ Fourth, if you are an existing practice, look at the historical way in which you have compensated physicians before you develop a new plan.

▶ Fifth, analyze alternatives, and sixth, make a recommendation for your practice. Once your partners reach consensus, take steps seven and eight, development of a transition process and implementation.

▶ Steps nine through eleven are ongoing: communicate the details of your plan, develop an appeals process, and revise the plan when circumstances change.

With respect to legal issues, anti-kickback, self-referral, corporate practice of medicine laws and other statutes govern physician compensation.[2] Seek legal guidance before you start your compensation project. Chapter 13 on Compliance contains relevant information.

EXHIBIT 8.8 Suggested goals for physician compensation plans

SUPPORT ACHIEVEMENT OF LONG-TERM PRACTICE OBJECTIVES	DISTRIBUTE CASH FAIRLY, CONSISTENTLY, AND APPROPRIATELY
▶ Ensure financial viability. ▶ Comply with relevant government laws and regulations. ▶ Promote harmony among the partners and between the partners and the entire workforce. ▶ Provide financial incentives for physician behavior that is consistent with the goals and philosophy of the practice. ▶ Acknowledge the competitive environment through benchmarking against industry standards. ▶ Support the practice's recognition of the importance of clinical performance, administrative work, participation in the healthcare community, provision of quality care, and workforce and patient satisfaction. ▶ Support physician recruitment and retention. ▶ Encourage the efficient and effective practice of medicine. ▶ Obtain and maintain credentials in your specialty. ▶ Recognize the desire of senior physicians who want to reduce their hours or become part-time employees.	▶ Distribute practice income in compliance with government regulations. ▶ Distribute practice income according to clinical effort, administrative contribution, documentation of quality care, continuing education, workforce satisfaction, patient satisfaction, and/or other factors that are important to your practice. ▶ Distribute cash in accordance with sources of revenue (e.g., managed care plans). ▶ Retain a portion of current earnings for future investment in the practice.

Your compensation plan should address two general goals, supporting your practice's long-term objectives and distributing cash fairly and appropriately. Exhibit 8.8 provides suggestions.

If you are an existing practice that is reviewing alternatives to your current compensation plan, obtain a good understanding of your historical and current methods. Educate yourself about the method(s) you use, a history of earnings for the entire practice and for individual physicians, unusual arrangements (e.g., unpaid working spouses, outside income, administrative compensation), your payer mix, individual physician performance, and the way in which you allocate overheads.

The basic methods of physician compensation are production formulas, salary formulas, capitation formulas, or a combination. Exhibit 8.9 explains how each method works and suggests some of the pros and cons, this exhibit can also be found on the website www. radcliffe-oxford.com/medicalpracticemanagement. If you would like detailed information on production formulas, Exhibit 8.10 lists resources available online from the American Academy of Family Practice (aafp.org) and the American College of Physicians (www. acponline.org/pmc).

EXHIBIT 8.9 Basic methods of physician compensation

COMPENSATION METHODOLOGY	FEATURES
Production formulas ("eat what you kill")	• Individual formulas reward physicians according to the revenue that each produces less the expenses allocated to each. • This method can result in lack of group perspective, potential disagreements over allocation, and micro-management of expenses. • Relative Value Units (RVUs) are often used to measure physician productivity.
Salary formulas	• Salaries are benchmarked against industry norms for a prescribed scope of work. Annual increases depend on merit and length of service. Lack of an incentive to work harder can be problematic. • Market-based salary and bonus plans strive to balance the stability of a salary with incentive payments linked to desired behaviors. These plans may include some features of production formulas.
Capitation formulas (if relevant in your market)	• Physicians are rewarded for the degree to which they meet the per member/ per month goals of managed care contracts. • Primary care physicians function as gatekeepers who manage care according to a fixed pre-paid budget.
Combination (2 examples)	• Example 1: the practice divides practice expenses equally among physicians and allocates revenue according to individual productivity. • This method is easy to calculate and understand. It promotes shared responsibility for costs and individual productivity. • This approach requires group agreement on percentage of income to be based on productivity vs base salary. • When physician use of resources varies widely, this method can be difficult to apply. • Example 2: Equal share formulas split the excess of revenue over expenses evenly among group members in order to reward teamwork. • Large variations in production, lack of incentives to work harder, and perception of inequities can be problematic.

EXHIBIT 8.10 Resources on production method of physician compensation

- American College of Physicians Practice Management Center (2003). "Income Distribution and Partner Buy-Ins". www.acponline.org/private/pmc/income_dist.pdf
- Moore, KJ (2002) "A Productivity Primer" www.aafp.org/fpm/20020500/72apro.html
- Moore, KJ (1999). "Bonus and Incentives – Three Key Questions" in Family Practice Management. www.aafp.org/fpm/990700fm/salaried.html

Regardless of which method(s) of compensation you select, make sure to address the following questions. How will compensation differ for partners and associates? Will you reward physicians for seniority? What non-clinical factors will you compensate, and at what rates? For example, if you encourage members of your practice to assume administrative responsibilities and/or participate in community healthcare activities, how will you pay for those activities? Will you reward business development as an incentive for physicians to see new patients? How will you pay for on-call? How will you allocate the cost of overhead items like administrative expenses, supplies, space, dedicated administrative support, and preferred office decorating? What benefit package will you offer to physicians?

Once you develop a compensation plan that is acceptable to your practice, review it regularly and revise it if necessary. Circumstances within and outside your practice will change, so don't think of your compensation method as cast in stone. Medical Group Management Association of America (MGMA), national search firms, and your professional association regularly survey practices throughout the country. You can purchase information that is relevant to your specialty to help you benchmark your own practice against industry standards.

Most important, communicate the details of your compensation plan to current members of your practice and to candidates that you recruit in the future. All physicians should understand exactly how it works. Finally, in spite of your best efforts, no system works perfectly. Develop a formal appeals process so that physicians can raise problems with the compensation system. Most practices ask the same group that worked on designing the compensation system to act as the board for appeals.

How Can You Develop a System for Evaluating Physician Performance?

Regardless of how you compensate the physicians in your practice, responsible management of your practice requires setting standards for physicians and measuring them regularly. Use your compensation method as a foundation for setting financial and non-financial standards. Exhibit 8.11 provides a framework for measuring physician work effort.

EXHIBIT 8.11 Suggested methods for measuring physician work effort

COMPONENTS	SOURCES OF INFORMATION
• Allocation of physician time between clinical work, call, administrative work, participation in committees, etc.	• Patient appointments kept
	• Physician-specific patients/enrollees by payer
• Number and % visits by physician adjusted by patient mix (e.g., age, complexity)	• Accounting records of billing/ collection by physician adjusted by payer

(continued)

COMPONENTS	SOURCES OF INFORMATION
▸ Billing/collection by physician adjusted by payer mix ▸ Number of patients/enrollees by physician, adjusted by patient and payer mix ▸ Hours worked by physician	▸ Information from PMS and/or EHR regarding patient mix

Based on suggestions by Gerald Benedict in *The Development and Management of Medical Groups.*[3]

Self-evaluation can be an effective way to monitor physicians' performance on non-financial factors. Exhibit 8.12 is a sample physician self-evaluation report and can also be found on the website www.radcliffe-oxford.com/medicalpracticemanagement.

EXHIBIT 8.12 Sample physician self-evaluation report

PHYSICIAN SELF-EVALUATION REPORT
PRACTICE NAME:
PHYSICIAN NAME: **DATE:**
Instructions: Please answer the following questions to help our practice evaluate physician performance. Return the completed form to Dr Swan, Managing Partner. Your responses will be kept confidential.
PATIENT CARE 1 How do you rate your provision of patient services and service quality? 2 With respect to clinical competence, rate your current skills and identify any areas in which you would like to improve. 3 Describe your interpersonal relationships with members of our workforce, with medical colleagues, and with staff at the hospital to which we admit patients. 4 During the past year, how have you promoted both our group and your own personal practice? 5 Describe your practice efficiency.
GOALS FOR IMPROVING PATIENT CARE Based on your answers to the questions above, what goals do you have for the coming year to improve your delivery of patient care? 1 _____ 2 _____ 3 _____
CONTINUING MEDICAL EDUCATION 1 List the CME activities in which you participated during the past year. List the meetings, the dates that you attended, and the CEU credits. 2 List any talks that you gave, papers that you wrote, or teaching duties that you performed during the year. 3 What are your plans for CME, talks, and papers for the coming year?

PHYSICIAN SELF-EVALUATION REPORT
ADMINISTRATIVE ACTIVITIES List all committees inside and outside our practice on which you served and your contributions to those committees.
COMMUNITY INVOLVEMENT 1   List any community organizations in which you have participated on behalf of our practice. Identify your responsibilities and contributions and the average amount of time/week that you have spent on this work. 2   Describe your involvement in regional healthcare activities on behalf of our practice. Identify your responsibilities and contributions and the average amount of time/week that you have spent on this work.
OTHER 1   List other outstanding contributions to our practice that are not mentioned above. 2   Identify physicians who have made an outstanding contribution to our practice and deserve special recognition. 3   Suggest ways in which our practice can better support you in your clinical, administrative, and community activities.
COMMENTS
Adapted from *The Physician Manager in Group Practice*[4] and from Flood SC, "Using Qualitative Self-Evaluation in Rating Physician Performance." May 1998. www.aafp.org/fpm/FPMprinter/980500fm/lead.html.

How Should You Handle Physician Departures from Your Practice?

Physician departures from your practice will occur for many reasons. Younger partners or salaried employees may seek other opportunities in a different location or a different size practice. Older partners who have been with the practice for many years may reduce their working hours or retire. You may decide to fire an employed physician for cause or buy out a physician's share in the partnership. You can't prevent these departures from happening, but you can take steps that discourage unwanted departures and that protect your practice when physicians leave.

Regardless of the cause for a physician departure from your practice, strive for civility by planning ahead. When you recruit and orient new physicians, clarify expectations, answer questions, and build protections into your legal documents. Be clear and complete in your explanations of job requirements, on-call, scheduling, administrative responsibilities, interpersonal relationships with physician and non-physician staff, community participation, professional education, compensation, opportunities for equity ownership, non-compete requirements upon termination, and tail coverage for malpractice insurance.

When a physician departure occurs, protect your practice by first checking with legal counsel and with your accountant. With their guidance, take the steps listed in Exhibit 8.13, this exhibit can also be found on the website www.radcliffe-oxford.com/medicalpracticemanagement.

EXHIBIT 8.13 Steps to take when physicians leave your practice

STEP	COMMENT
Review all documents that should have been signed when the physician joined your practice.	▶ Check the employment agreement, shareholders' agreement or operating agreement, and deferred compensation arrangement. ▶ Review advance notice requirements, retirement plan details, and non-compete covenants. ▶ Determine whether or not the departure requires return of recruitment and relocation payments. ▶ Ask your accountant if there are tax implications with deferred compensation agreements.
Review your practice's policies for departure of employees.	▶ Take the same steps for departing physicians that you do for departing employees regarding returning keys, changing computer passwords, terminating remote computer access, changing entry codes, and returning all forms and manuals.
Develop a plan to notify patients.	▶ Check your state's requirements requiring written notification and other issues. ▶ Word your communication tactfully. Even if the circumstances of the departure are negative, be positive with patients. ▶ Be consistent. Your workforce, written letters, and messages on your telephone system should say the same thing and provide clear instructions to patients.
Develop a plan to notify providers in the community.	▶ As with communications to patients, strive for tact and consistency. ▶ Remember that providers in your community who are friends with the departing physician may take sides and stop referring business to your practice.
Review advance notice provisions of the contract with the departing physician.	▶ Make sure that the departing physician provides the required advance notice. Apply penalties if he/she doesn't.
Review the retirement plan.	▶ Check eligibility and vesting requirements carefully.
Address tail coverage.	▶ The departing physician or the practice should purchase tail coverage to cover malpractice claims made after the physician's departure. ▶ Tail coverage is expensive but very important to risk management. Don't ignore it.
Clarify ownership of the patient chart and other demographic information.	▶ The practice, not the departing physician, owns the patient record. ▶ Most states allow patients to request that the chart be forwarded to the departing physician. ▶ In some but not all states, you can charge for copies of the records.
Pay attention to the HIPAA Privacy and Security Rules.	▶ Make sure you don't violate these rules by sharing patient information without appropriate safeguards.
Schedule departures with patient needs in mind.	▶ Make sure you provide care for patients who need it, especially if the needs are anticipated (e.g., deliveries).
Protect your practice from solicitation of existing employees by the departing physician.	▶ Most contracts address this issue.

Based on Wall JD. *A Must-Do List for the Departing Physician.* 2005. www.aafp.org/fpm/FPMprinter/20051000/54amus.html

Where Can You Learn More about the Physician Issues Discussed in this Chapter?

Good resources on issues discussed in this chapter are listed below:

▶ American Academy of Physician Assistants website (www.aapa.org).

▶ American College of Nurse Practitioners website (www.nurse.org/acnp).

▶ Benedict, GS (1996). The Development and Management of Medical Groups. Englewood, CO. Medical Group Management Association of America.

▶ Bode, GL (2000). "An Economic 'Report Card" for Physicians" in The Business of Medical Practice. New York, Springer Publishing Company, Inc.

▶ Hekman, KM (2002). Physician Compensation Models for Aligning Financial Goals and Incentives, 2nd Edition. Englewood, CO. Medical Group Management Association of America.

▶ Krill, MA (1995). Successful Partnerships for the Future: Administrator–Physician Dynamics. Englewood, CO. Medical Group Management Association of America.

▶ Medical Group Management Association of America (MGMA) Surveys and Other Reports:
  — Income Distribution – Call Coverage
  — Income Distribution – Expense Allocation
  — Income Distribution – Incentive Plan
  — Income Distribution – Relative Value Units
  — MGMA Physician Compensation and Production Survey: 2005 Report Based on 2004 Data
  — MGMA Management Compensation Survey: 2005 Report Based on 2004 Data
  — Physicians – Benefits
  — Physician Employment Contracts
  — Physician Orientation
  — Physician Performance Appraisal
  — Physician Satisfaction Survey

▶ Micklitsch CN and Ryan-Mitylng TA (1996). Physician Performance Management: Tool for Survival and Success. Englewood, CO. Medical Group Management Association of America.

▶ Silver JK (1998). The Business of Medicine. Philadelphia, PA. Hanley & Belfus, Inc.

▶ Zaslove M (1998). The Successful Physician: A Productivity Handbook for Practitioners. Englewood, CO. Medical Group Management Association of America.

References

1   Berger-Fiffy J. How to Find the Perfect Job. In: Silver JK, editor. *The Business of Medicine.* Philadelphia, PA: Hanley & Belfus, Inc.; 1998.
2   Moore KJ. Bonuses and Incentives: Three Key Questions. July/August 1999 Family Practice Management; 1999. (www.aafp.org/fpm/FPMprinter/990700fm/salaried.html).

3   Benedict G. *The Development and Management of Medical Groups.* Englewood, CO: Medical Group Management Association; 1996.

4   Pollard J. *The Physician Manager in Group Practice.* Englewood, CO: Medical Group Management Association of America; 1995.

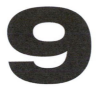 # Using Outsourcing Effectively

Now that you know the scope of medical practice management and have divided managerial responsibilities among physicians and your practice administrator/manager, you can well understand that it may make good sense to outsource one or more functions to an external consultant with particular expertise. You may lack the internal expertise to handle particular tasks. If you are a small practice, you and your staff may be so involved with daily practice operations that it's unrealistic for you to take on new and complicated projects like HIPAA Privacy and Security Rule compliance, renegotiation of managed care contracts, and innovations in information technology.

This section will address the following questions:

▶ What functions should you consider outsourcing to external experts?

▶ What problems can outsourcing help you address, and what are the advantages and disadvantages of outsourcing?

▶ If you decide to outsource any of the functions identified in this chapter, how should you select a consultant or vendor?

Please note that Chapter 10 also contains general information on working with consultants, so you may want to read that material too.

What Functions Should You Consider Outsourcing?

You can outsource a variety of the managerial responsibilities in your practice to experts outside your practice who handle particular functions and who are directly accountable to someone in your practice. Functions that practices commonly outsource are managed care, billing and collections, information technology, human resources, and financial planning.

Managed Care

Most physicians and practice administrator/managers would be happy if managed care would disappear. In general, they hate it, avoid it, and rarely devote the attention that it warrants given its impact on the financial health of their medical practices. For the time being, however, managed care is an integral part of the American healthcare system. If you don't want to handle this important responsibility internally, consider outsourcing it to a practice management consultant. Here are some of the problems that outsourcing can address:

‣ As a result of staff turnover and inattention to detail, many practices don't know what managed care contracts they have in place, the most recent renegotiation dates, or the amount of the reimbursement they should be receiving from payers. If you are not familiar with your existing contracts, you can't determine if the situation is favourable or unfavourable for your practice.

‣ Although most states require payers to provide medical practices with CPT-code specific reimbursement for some or all codes, many practices don't realize they must request this information. Without knowing what they should be paid, they can't compare their actual reimbursement with the contractual expectation.

‣ Although payers do occasionally change their fees for all participating providers in particular specialties, in general, they don't contact medical practices and offer to increase reimbursement. If you want an increase, you have to request one.

‣ Each managed care plan has a unique method of reimbursement. Some pay a fixed percentage of Medicare, but not all plans relate this percentage to the same Medicare year. Other plans use proprietary fee schedules. In some but not all parts of the country, capitation arrangements are common. Because there are so many variations in reimbursement, practices find it difficult to compare reimbursement across plans.

‣ It would be nice to think that all physicians receive the same reimbursement for the same level of service, but that's not how managed care works. The size and location of your practice and your importance in the networks in which you participate are all contributing factors.

By outsourcing your managed care work to an external consultant who reviews both rates and contract language, you may gain the following advantages:

‣ Consultants that represent multiple clients have developed good working relationships with the different managed care plans. They know whom to contact at each plan. More important, they know how to frame a request for a rate increase in a way that is most likely to produce a favorable result for your practice.

‣ Contract language review is a tedious task. You must read not only the legal agreement, but also information that is contained in detailed administrative manuals and on each plan's website. Consultants with experience in reviewing and organizing this information into an easily understandable format can save you hours of reading and analysis.

‣ Depending on your selection of a managed care consultant, you can engage someone who is willing to teach your staff what to do. Once you learn the steps, you can decide whether or not you want the consultant to do all of your managed care contracts or if you would like your staff to assume ongoing responsibility for the work.

If you decide to outsource your managed care work, make sure you ask appropriate questions in making your selection. Exhibit 9.1 provides guidance.

EXHIBIT 9.1 Questions to ask potential managed care consultants

QUESTION	COMMENTS
What is your experience with managed care contract review and rate negotiations?	Identify an experienced consultant who has dealt with different plans in your community.
What kind of practices has the consultant represented?	Select a consultant with experience in your particular specialty.
Will the consultant work on some but not all of your managed care contracts if that is your preference?	Some managed care consultants will only work for clients that authorize them to work on all managed care contracts. You may not want the consultant to do all this work; don't pay for what you don't need.
Will the consultant teach someone in your practice what to do?	Find a consultant who will explain to your practice exactly what he/she is doing. You may continue to outsource the work, but you should know what is being done.
How will the consultant charge for the service?	Most consultants charge a flat fee/managed care contract or an hourly rate. Either is fine. Make sure you know the terms of your arrangement.
Check references.	Ask references whether or not they were satisfied with the consultant's work. For anti-trust reasons, do not ask references about the amount of financial gain the consultant brought to the practice.

Billing and Collections

The term revenue cycle management describes all of the steps required to bill and collect revenue for the services that you provide to patients (see Chapter 6). The word "cycle" is important for several reasons. First, success often requires repetition of the same steps in a cyclical fashion until you are finally reimbursed the proper amount. Cycle also applies to the workflow process within your practice. Collecting accurate patient demographic information at the registration point affects your ability to submit a clean claim following patient check-out. Finally, cycle also applies to all that you need to do before you even see a patient – i.e., set your fees at an appropriate level, negotiate your managed care contracts so you receive reasonable reimbursement and make sure that your billing and collections processes support your effort. Many practices struggle with the billing and collections portion of revenue cycle management. Here are common problems:

- The individual responsible for billing and collections is not knowledgeable about this very critical area for all medical practices. Sometimes the practice administrator/manager supervises the billing and collections functions even though he/she does not have the background and experience to identify and resolve problems. When issues arise, they remain unresolved.

- Billing and collections, particularly collections, can be an unpleasant job for those who dislike dealing with people and listening to their problems. High staff turnover is common. If you are spending money to recruit, hire, and train billing and collections staff, only to find that within a very short time you have to do the same thing all over again, outsourcing may be a good alternative.

- Success in billing and collections requires focus and concentration. In many small practices where the staff multi-task, there's no standardization in the billing and collection processes. When staff have time, they work on an unpaid claim or two with little regard to the dollar value or days outstanding of the outstanding claims.

▶ Success in collecting from different managed care plans requires the ability to develop good working relationships with specific individuals at each plan who understand your practice. Your staff should also know how to use online claims checking services that most plans make available to participating providers. You want your staff to get claims paid. If your employees tell you that they have made a call and nobody called back, you have a problem.

▶ Self-pay by patients is becoming more and more important to all practices. Employers are shifting the burden of health insurance to employees, and some are now opting for health savings accounts. Many people who are between jobs or self-employed may have no health insurance at all. Some practices may have a longstanding tradition of not asking patients for money, and staff may have trouble making the transition to a different procedure that requires payment at the time of service.

If you are considering outsourcing your billing and collections, be aware of the advantages and disadvantages. Here are the advantages:

▶ You may reduce your accounts receivable and generate more revenue sooner than you are currently doing.

▶ Within your practice, you can focus on clinical care, not billing and collections.

▶ You'll have access to experts in coding, management, and insurance who will focus on these tasks. Other pressing operational needs will not divert them as they would in-house staff who are multi-tasking.

▶ Staff turnover and the accompanying costs of recruiting, hiring, and training new staff may decrease.

▶ As the owner of your practice, you may have more, not less, control over billing and collections than you would if these functions are dependent on in-house personnel who lack expertise and/or who keep leaving your practice.

▶ You can free up space in your office that was previously occupied by billing hardware.

▶ You can reduce the number of phone calls about billing and collections that come directly to your practice. Billing and collections companies answer the phone with your practice name, so patients do not realize that they are talking with people outside your office.

▶ You can increase the hours of coverage for answering questions about billing and collections.

Outsourcing billing and collections can have two disadvantages to your practice. Your practice administrator/manager and/or billing staff may feel threatened by the change. If, however, the decision to outsource gives your practice administrator/manager more time to focus on other projects, he/she may welcome the change. You may be able to assign the billing staff to other responsibilities. A second disadvantage to your practice may be the perception that you are losing control over receivables. If you provide guidance and feedback to the outsourcing company, however, you'll retain control. Exhibit 9.2 describes the experience of an internal medicine practice that had a very good experience with outsourcing billing and collections.

EXHIBIT 9.2 Empire Medical Associates' experience with outsourced billing and collections

Empire Medical Associates was an internal medical practice that experienced a difficult transition from a hospital-owned to a private practice. Once the practice left the large management structure of the hospital, it had to hire new billing staff and create a new billing cycle. The group attempted to hire well-qualified individuals to run its in-house billing department. Unfortunately, the billing department did not thrive. The practice manager lacked the knowledge and experience that was necessary to provide supervision. The relationship between billing and the front office was hostile. When the accounts receivable escalated to more than $600,000, the practice had to decide whether to create a new billing department or outsource the function to an external company.

Empire decided that it could not afford to make more mistakes in the management of billing and collections. It interviewed several billing and collections companies and selected one that specialized in small practices. Within a year after the outsourcing decision, the receivables decreased and the billing company exceeded its benchmarks for collections. The cost to the practice of outsourcing billing and collections was less than the cost of maintaining this function within the practice.

If you would like to explore outsourcing your billing and collections, review the vendor questions listed in Exhibit 9.3. This exhibit can also be found on the website www.radcliffe-oxford.com/medicalpracticemanagement.

EXHIBIT 9.3 Questions to ask billing and collections vendors

QUESTION	COMMENTS
What is the ownership structure of the vendor?	Is the vendor independently owned or a subsidiary of another organization?
What is the vendor's history and long-range strategic plan?	Look for both stability and clear future direction.
How does the vendor service new clients?	Will current or new staff be assigned to your practice?
What is the vendor's attitude toward practices of your size and specialty?	Some vendors are only interested in large practices; make sure you will be a priority.
What practice management system does the vendor use?	▸ Most vendors will want you to use the same practice management system as they use. This requirement may mean a change for you – or not. ▸ Determine if the vendor that provides your electronic health record can and is willing to interface with the practice management system.
Check vendor references.	Call the references and make one or more site visits to current clients.
What is the vendor's set-up?	Visit the vendor's site, meet with the staff there, and develop a sense of the level of professionalism.

(continued)

QUESTION	COMMENTS
Who will manage your account?	Make sure you are comfortable with the individual assigned to handle your account. Reserve the right to ask for a change.
How does the vendor charge clients?	Ask if the vendor charges a percentage of net collections or a flat monthly fee. Obtain the fees for software licensing, set-up, hardware, and connectivity.
What staff training will the vendor provide at the outset and throughout your relationship?	Make sure the vendor provides training at the outset and on an ongoing basis. Make sure you know which portions of this training are included in your purchase price and which portions are additional.
Will the vendor help you clean up past claims that are more than 90 days old?	Some vendors won't clean up old claims. Others will do so for an additional fee.
Given your particular set of circumstances, what savings does the vendor expect to recognize?	Your vendor's estimate of return on investment will depend on your ability to provide valid information on your current situation.
What are the details of the transition process and how long will it take?	Obtain specific information, and make sure you understand if you will be running dual systems for any length of time.
How frequently will the vendor meet with your practice?	Make sure the vendor will meet with you regularly. No matter how good your choice of vendor may be, ongoing communication is essential.
What reports will the vendor provide on a regular basis?	Make sure you will receive clear and regular reports that will help both you and the vendor take corrective action.

Information Technology

Information technology (IT) is rapidly becoming a critical component of practice management. Physicians who have recently completed their training and are setting up practices are thinking about ways in which information technology can help them keep their overhead expenses low. Physicians who are already in practice and who are dependent on paper records and systems are learning how their practice management system (PMS), electronic health records (EHR), e-prescribing, website, and the integration among these applications can help them deliver higher quality and more efficient care. The handwriting is already on the wall. In the years to come, both public and private payers will continue to put in place financial incentives to support the growing acceptance of information technology applications. You must make good decisions about products, interconnectivity, ongoing IT support, and compliance with the HIPAA Privacy and Security Rules.

Unfortunately, many practices approach IT planning and implementation in haphazard ways. They often begin by looking at the products on the market, rather than by assessing their own needs. Seduced by the bells and whistles that they see at trade shows and that vendors promote, they skip the IT planning phase and rush to purchase systems or packages that turn out to be unsuitable for their particular practice. Another cause for poor IT decisions is reliance on internal staff who enjoy using computers but who are poorly informed about current trends, external regulations, interconnectivity, proposals, and contracts. Still another source of trouble is seeking inexpensive or free advice from friends and relatives. Remember the saying – "You Get What You Pay For." Exhibit 9.4 describes the experience of Brown Street Internal Medicine.

EXHIBIT 9.4 Brown Street Family Medicine's EHR experience

Dr Jones opened Brown Street Family Medicine when he bought his practice back from the academic medical center that had owned it. He loved information technology. Without input from his staff, he quickly purchased an EHR system that a local vendor had developed. The system didn't work well, and so he purchased a second system. That system also didn't work, and Dr Jones went back to his original vendor. Dr Jones wasted both time and money because he didn't plan carefully and involve his staff.

There's great value in asking an external IT consultant to help you plan, purchase, implement, and evaluate your information technology options. You'll learn a great deal that you don't currently know, and you'll probably get a better result than if you dabble in an area in which you are not an expert.

Exhibit 9.5 contains a checklist for interviewing potential IT consultants and can also be found on the website www.radcliffe-oxford.com/medicalpracticemanagement.

EXHIBIT 9.5 Checklist for interviewing potential IT consultants

QUESTION	COMMENTS
How long have you provided IT support services for medical practices?	You are looking for a company with experience with medical practices; general IT experience isn't good enough.
How many medical and dental clients do you currently support?	The number of clients will help you evaluate business growth and stability.
What are your future plans for growth and expansion?	Select a consultant with a serious business strategy, not one that dabbles in helping people with their computers.
How do you recruit, train, and retain staff?	You want an IT consultant that has a strategy for hiring and keeping qualified individuals.
What is the size of your payroll, and how do you add people when you need help for a specific project?	Make sure that the IT consultant you select has the capacity to handle new clients.
What certifications do your employees have?	Look for staff with appropriate qualifications, not people who enjoy computers.
What specific services do you provide for hardware and software?	Ask about assistance with hardware and software selection, guidance for security, assistance and training with various software programs, ability to interface applications that you may have purchased from different vendors.
How do you respond to typical inquiries from medical practice clients?	Ask about response time off-site versus on-site assistance, documentation about requests for assistance.
How do you charge for your services?	Most IT consultants charge hourly or flat monthly rates. Check to see if there is a special after-hours rate.
Do you have service performance goals for your staff?	Service to your practice will be as good as the staff; check on the expectations that the vendor sets for its own staff.
Who can the practice call for references?	Ask the references if they received the product and service that they expected to receive.

Human Resources

Your employees are your most important assets. Recruiting, hiring, firing, supervising, training, doing regular performance evaluations, making sure you comply with state and federal law, reviewing your benefit package, and upgrading your salary scales are some of the tasks you should be doing on a regular basis. If you are like most practices with 15 or fewer physicians, you don't have the internal expertise that you need, and work on these tasks takes time away from pressing clinical responsibilities. Traditionally, physicians have delegated the human resources tasks to a practice administrator/manager.

Here's a list of the human resources problems that medical practices frequently encounter:

▶ Many practices lack systematic ways to perform routine human resources functions, so they treat employees inconsistently. Staff complain about favoritism. Different standards regarding work expectations, performance evaluations, and other issues apply to different people.

▶ The practice administrator/manager has been promoted from within the practice, and he/she is uncomfortable supervising and reviewing co-workers who were once peers.

▶ Physicians are inexperienced and uncomfortable with employee performance evaluations. They postpone the reviews or don't do them at all. Employees crave feedback and become frustrated and uncooperative when they don't receive it.

If you would like to explore external assistance for one or more of your human resource tasks, you have three options. First, you can engage a consultant to help you with one or more projects. For example, you can ask a consultant to help you develop and implement a performance evaluation system. You may already outsource your payroll function. Second, you can outsource multiple human resource tasks to the same vendor in what is known as business processing outsourcing (BPO). Third, you can go one step further than the BPO approach and partner with a professional employer organization (PEO). With the third option, your employees are actually on the payroll of the PEO and you "lease" them back.

Each of these three options has advantages and disadvantages. Here's a list of advantages that you may recognize if you select the third option, the PEO:

▶ You have access to professionally trained and experienced human resource experts. They save you time and money so you and your staff can concentrate on revenue generation, profitability, and quality improvement.

▶ You can offer a richer benefit package to your employees than you can as a small and perhaps solo employer. The PEO's "workforce" is larger than your own, and this leverage allows the purchase of more and better types of health and dental insurance, disability insurance, retirement packages, and other benefits.

▶ When your employees need counseling and/or coaching to better improve their job performance, experts can provide these services.

▶ The PEO's professional staff can answer questions about benefits more quickly and accurately than you can.

▶ The PEO develops the documentation that you need in your practice: your Employee Handbook, forms, policies, and procedures.

▶ You can reduce the risk to your practice by gaining access to professional advice on employment-related issues.

As with all outsourcing, there is always a downside. If you outsource your human resources to a PEO, you share, not relinquish, control of your employees.

If you would like to investigate outsourcing your human resources to a PEO, BPO, or other external consultant, ask the questions listed in Exhibit 9.6.

EXHIBIT 9.6 Questions for a PEO, BPO, or other external HR consultant

Questions

▶ How long has the organization/individual been in business?

▶ What are the organization/individual's future plans?

▶ If you are talking to a PEO, does the entity have a license in the state where it is operating?

▶ If you are talking to a PEO, is it accredited by the appropriate professional organization (e.g., Employer Service Assurance Corporation)?

▶ Who manages your account?

▶ How does the organizational/individual involve specific experts as needed?

▶ What do references say about the organization/individual?

Financial Planning

Just as physicians develop a diagnosis and treatment plan for their patients, they should put in place a financial plan for themselves as individuals and for their practice. If you are thinking about the long-term, checking monthly information from your accountant is not enough; you need to think ahead (Interview by author with Karen Diamond and Ed Barber, Merrill Lynch, 2005).

Since physicians are comfortable with research related to patient care, they often assume that they should apply their skills to their own investments. Sometimes they "self treat" so they don't have to pay an outside advisor. Or, they may feel that they know more than professional financial advisors. Financial professionals have another name for such an approach; they call it "financial malpractice." From their perspective, the patient/physician is prescribing a treatment without fully understanding what ails him/her.

When you seek outside help with financial planning, here are some important suggestions:

▶ *Educate yourself.* An excellent resource is William B. Howard's chapter, "Planning for Your Personal Financial Success," in JK Silver's book.[1]

▶ *Get organized* by bringing together the items you'll need for financial planning. Howard suggests that you document cash and equivalents, notes receivable, securities, limited partnerships, insurance contracts, personal assets, liabilities, retirement plans, and tax, personal, and business documents.[1]

▶ *Plan first, and then invest.* The person who helps you with financial planning may or may not be the same individual who makes or facilitates the investments. Some physicians prefer an independent financial planner who has no relationship to the investments, even if this approach means two fees. Another approach is to ask the same firm to provide both planning and investment advice. Some but not all advisors in large firms are trained to do both. The advice is free, and the advisors earn their fees from the investments. The advantage to this approach is that the advice can be ongoing as your needs and circumstances change.

▶ *Check the credentials* of the financial advisor(s). Is he or she a Certified Financial Planner (CFP)? The CFP designation is earned after many hours of training, studying, and intensive testing in all areas of financial planning and investments.

▶ *Don't be put off by fees.* You don't work for free and neither do financial planning professionals. Remember the old adage, "You get what you pay for." Many fees are hidden, so the average investor thinks he or she is getting something for nothing. Variable annuities are a good example. The insurance company markets the product as having no annual fee, but in fact, the mutual funds within the annuity may charge between 1% and 5% annually as expenses and management fees. Investors can't see the fees because they are deducted from performance. Annuities aren't bad; just don't think that they are free.

▶ *Stay involved* with your financial plan and investments, but don't do them yourself unless you are sure you know what you are doing. Meet with your financial advisor at least twice each year for a financial check-up. Regular topics of discussion should be your risk tolerance, investment objectives, asset allocation, portfolio performance vs the indices, and your cash flow needs. Rebalance your portfolio periodically to take advantage of changing trends in the economy. Make tax management part of the overview; your financial advisor can work collaboratively with your CPA and attorney. Your advisor may also be able to help you with insurance needs.

▶ *Don't postpone establishing a retirement plan* for your practice because you don't want to make contributions for your employees. In the end, you will be hurt more by not taking advantage of one of the best retirement investment opportunities.

▶ *Remember the parallels between medicine and financial management.* Planning and investing goes way beyond selecting the right stock or bond. It is about having someone who acts like your primary care physician by diagnosing your problem, calling in the specialists, and coordinating your care. Call it the holistic approach to financial management.

References

1   Howard WB. Planning for Your Personal Financial Success. In: Silver JK, *The Business of Medicine*. Philadelphia: Hanley & Belfus, Inc; 1998.

10 Hiring and Managing Consultants

At one time or another, most medical practices will hire an external consultant to help them start or improve their organizations. Chapter 9 identified functions that physicians often outsource to consultants: managed care contract review and rate negotiation, human resources, information technology, and financial planning. Depending on your internal resources, you may have other needs for external help.

This chapter addresses the following questions:

- When you hire a consultant, what should you do ahead of time to make sure you find an individual and/or firm that is right for you?
- What are the general characteristics of a good consultant?
- How do you find a good consultant?
- How do you start?
- After you have interviewed several candidates, what are the next steps?
- How do consultants charge for their services?
- What should be in the written agreement that you have with your consultant?

What Should You Do Before You Hire A Consultant?

Medical practices call in an external consultant when they have organizational, financial, marketing, or other issues that they can't or don't want to handle themselves. They frequently forget that the first step in getting good help is the practice's own responsibility – describing the problem.

As the owner of your practice, organize your own thoughts and solicit input from your partners and staff. What is the history of your practice? What is your current status and where do you want to be in five years? What is your management structure, and are responsibilities clear? How well are the people in key positions performing their jobs? What problem(s) do you want the consultant to help you solve? Why haven't you solved the problem(s) yourselves? Do you lack the time, knowledge, staff time, or all three? What would you like a consultant to accomplish for you? Do you have a budget and a time frame? What role do you want to play in working with a consultant?

The more carefully you address each of these questions, the better able you will be to explain to the consultants whom you interview exactly what you want to accomplish. Your clarity can enhance the likelihood of receiving a proposal for consulting services that meets your needs and budgetary limits. Exhibit 10.1 describes a practice that asked for help with a problematic practice manager.

EXHIBIT 10.1 Tall Oaks ObGyn – from the consultant's perspective

Tall Oaks ObGyn engaged a practice management consultant for advice on disciplining its practice manager, a woman from the billing department whom they had promoted and who was now having trouble managing more than 20 employees. Here's what the consultant discovered. Thirty-five years ago, four physicians founded the practice. The founding partners had strong working relationships with each other and with their staff. When the founding partners retired, four new physicians replaced them. By default, one of those physicians acted as the Managing Partner, but as a group, the four partners had very different ideas about practice management. The practice manager received different and contradictory directions from each of the four physicians. She was unclear about her job responsibilities and accountability. When the consultant finished talking with all the physicians and employees in the practice, he realized that the physicians had misidentified the problem. They themselves were as much a problem as their practice manager.

What are the General Characteristics of a Good Consultant?

Regardless of the project for which you are seeking advice, there are general characteristics of a good consultant. Look for training and experience in the particular area for which you need help, and, more important, look at the consultant's approach to the work and to you as the client.

With respect to training and experience, education, professional credentials, and previous consulting experience are all important. It is less important to hire someone who has done precisely what you want done than it is to hire an individual with a track record of learning and client service.

Learn about a consultant's approach to his/her clients and projects by asking many questions. Here are some suggestions.

‣ How does the consultant characterize his/her relationships with clients? Some consultants tell you that they solve problems *for* their clients. Others describe long-term relationships with clients that imply client *dependency* on the consultant. Still others talk about themselves as *coaches or mentors* who *collaborate* with clients to help the clients find the answers. Unless you want to engage the consultant on a long-term retainer, look for a coach/mentor.[1]

‣ How does the consultant approach a new client with a new problem? Each practice is unique, so avoid hiring someone who brings the same solution to every set of circumstances. Probe for willingness to learn about your processes and organizational culture. Do you detect a keen interest in problem-solving? You want a consultant who can apply his/her education and experience to your unique situation.

‣ Look for objectivity. You are hiring outside help because you want an objective look at your practice. You don't want someone who echoes what you say for fear of displeasing you.

‣ How does the consultant prioritize work? Can you be sure that your project will receive the attention that it needs? Ask how the consultant organizes his/her time and projects so you don't find your practice at the bottom of long list of unfinished work.

▸ Who will do the work on your project? Ask each consultant if he/she does the work. Some consultants delegate projects or components of projects to junior staff members or to colleagues with whom they contract. If they do, they should let you know before they begin the work.

▸ What does the consultant do when he/she doesn't have the expertise that is needed? In many projects, something comes up that the individual consultant or consulting organization can't handle. Engage a consultant who is comfortable saying "I don't know" or "I don't do that," and who has a network of colleagues who can help.

How Do You Find a Good Consultant?

Consultants depend on their reputations, so ask your medical colleagues if they know anyone who can help. Also check with your state and local medical societies; these organizations can give you the names of several individuals and organizations in your particular geographic area. You can of course check the Internet, but that approach is less effective than word of mouth. After you get recommendations from reliable sources, check the consultant websites.

How Do You Start?

Your first step is to contact the consultant by phone and ask general questions about areas of expertise, availability, and price. Your time is valuable, so if someone cannot do what you need, is not available, or is out of your price range, stop right there and look for an alternative.

After you have identified at least two consultants that can potentially provide help, set up face-to-face informational meetings. Ask other partners and/or your practice administrator/manager to participate. Use the time to exchange information. You have not yet engaged the consultant, so you are looking for good personal chemistry, not solutions. Describe what is going on at your practice and ask the consultant the questions listed earlier in this chapter.

What Steps Do You Take Next?

Once you have identified at least two consulting candidates, ask each one for a proposal. Specify exactly what you want the proposals to contain so you can make a valid comparison. Ask for a statement of the problem(s), a description of the consultant's approach, a list of tasks, a proposed timetable, a budget, deliverables, clarification of what you as the client will be expected to do, and references. If you are dealing with a large consulting organization, make sure you know who will do the work. As explained above, a partner or other senior person may make the initial call and then assign the work to a junior person. If that is the plan, you should know in advance and make sure that you have the opportunity to meet the individual who will work directly with you. See Appendix G, Exhibit G.1, which can be found on the website www.radcliffe-oxford.com/medicalpracticemanagement, for a sample proposal for consulting services.

Once you have received two proposals, compare and contrast them with each other. Call the references. If you have unanswered questions, call the consultants for clarification. Based on the results of your calls and your evaluation of the proposals, make your decision.

How Do Consultants Charge for their Services?

Consultants generally charge a fixed fee or an hourly rate for their services. If the consultant can confidently estimate the number of hours for a project and give you a fixed rate, that approach is less financially risky for you. It is not always possible to predict the amount of time a project will take. For example, if you engage a consultant to help you with managed care, review of the contract documents, administrative manuals, and information available on the plan website is predictable. Less predictable is the amount of time that will be needed for negotiations to reach an outcome that is satisfactory to your practice and to the managed care plans. In this type of situation, you could pay the consultant a fee that is partially fixed and partially variable.

Be sure to ask about billing for travel time and expenses. Consultants have different policies. Some don't charge for travel time when the client is located within a particular geographic radius. Others always charge for travel time. Particularly at times when gas prices escalate, check this item ahead of time.

Also ask about rate increases. If you are entering into a relationship that you expect to extend for more than a year, make sure you and the consultant are in agreement on the process for rate increases. A reasonable protection is sixty days' written notice to you with your written acceptance of the changes.

Most consultants require a non-refundable up-front payment of a portion of the total estimated fee. This amount is applied to the project, and is not an addition to the project fee. Your willingness to make this first payment assures the consultant that you are committed to go forward with the work.

In general, consultants send monthly invoices. Request a progress report with each invoice so you know exactly what the consultant has accomplished and if there are any problems.

What Should an Agreement for Consulting Services Contain?

The Agreement for Consulting Services is the legal contract between your practice and the consultant. After you and the consultant have agreed on the scope of work, timing, and other details, you can incorporate this information into the formal Agreement. See Appendix G, Exhibit G.2 for a sample Agreement for Consulting Services. Appendix G can be found on the website www.radcliffe-oxford.com/medicalpracticemanagement.

References

1   Carucci RA, Tetenbaum TJ. *The Value-Creating Consultant*. New York: American Management Association; 2000.

11 Quality of Care

Not so long ago, the aura that surrounded the medical profession could be summed up in one short phrase: "I'm a physician, trust me." Practicing medicine in the twenty-first century, however, will require more than trust. Patients and society will say to physicians, "Yes, we trust you, but show us the data."[1] Physicians will be expected to demonstrate the following core competencies: provision of patient care, knowledge, interpersonal and communication skills, professionalism, practice-based learning, and system-based practice. (Paul Miles, MD. Speech to Alice Aycock Poe Center for Health Education. May, 2005. Interview by author. July, 2005.) Every practicing physician must be able to ask and answer two important questions:
1   How do I know that what I'm doing works?
2   How can I improve what I do?

For most physicians, quality and quality improvement are not high priorities. A 2003 Commonwealth Fund Survey of Quality of Care covering more than 1800 physicians throughout the country confirmed this observation.[2] The study's authors found that physicians' adoption of measures, tools, and quality is moving slowly and is not where it should be to achieve a high performance. A major obstacle to physicians' making quality improvement routine was lack of information about their own practices. The study also noted that physicians are uncomfortable sharing physician-specific performance data with the general public, with their patients, or with medical leadership. Finally, the study observed that practice size affects the likelihood that physicians receive and use data on quality of care. Those in practices with 50 or more physicians were more likely to be involved in quality improvement activities than those in smaller practices.

This chapter will address the following questions:
▶ What are quality and quality improvement?
▶ What quality and quality improvement initiatives already exist?
▶ How can you use measurement to compare your current status with post-improvement status?
▶ If you want to make quality of care and quality improvement a priority for your practice, what steps should you take?

Appendix H, which can be found on the website www.radcliffe-oxford.com/medical practicemanagement, contains additional information to help you implement a quality improvement program: a glossary of terms related to quality; national public and private agencies, organizations, and associations that are focusing on healthcare quality and improvement; recommended books and articles; opportunities for continuing education on quality and quality improvement; online information related to the promotion of quality in healthcare; and Programs in the Centers for Medicare & Medicaid Services (CMS) Physician Focused Quality Initiative.

What Are Quality and Quality Improvement in Healthcare?

The Institute of Medicine (IOM) defines quality as "the degree to which health services for individuals and populations increase the likelihood of desired health outcomes and are consistent with current professional knowledge."[3] The IOM's important 1991 report, *Crossing the Quality Chasm. A New Health System for the 21st Century*,[4] extends this concept a step further and comments: "Americans should be able to count on receiving care that meets their needs and is based on the best scientific knowledge." Quality is the difference between the care that is given now and the care that could be delivered, given what we already know. As the IOM report documents thoroughly, Americans don't have that guarantee, and the difference between what exists now and the ideal is a chasm, not merely a gap.

The quality chasm in healthcare isn't large because healthcare professionals don't know enough or try hard enough. Even the major deficiency in the American healthcare financing system – payment for services, not for care – is not the primary culprit. Outmoded systems of work are the major barrier that prevents all Americans from receiving state-of-the-art healthcare. In setting an agenda to address this system malfunction, the Institute of Medicine calls for healthcare that is safe, effective, patient-centered, timely, efficient, and equitable.

The evaluation of quality of care should focus on structure, process, and outcomes.[5] Structural quality refers to the health system capabilities of both large and small systems. Process quality looks at clinician/patient interactions. Outcomes evaluation refers to changes in health status. Although it is possible to measure the quality of structure, process, and outcome, most quality of care information is about appropriateness and professional standards.[4]

Just where does quality improvement fit in? Quality improvement is the method for closing the gap between the current state(s) and the desirable state(s), using measurement before, during, and after to track changes and results. Improvement science is a formal body of knowledge that applies the scientific method to improving complex systems. The principles of improvement science involve:[6]

1 Understanding healthcare as a system
2 Using a balanced set of process and outcome measures tracked over time to determine if change results in improvement
3 Using an explicit evidence base to determine which changes should be implemented and tested
4 Focusing on multidisciplinary teams to make change
5 Avoiding a focus only on poor performers.

The IOM recommends six steps for bringing both the American healthcare system as a whole and its many components toward a place that will give every individual the care that he or she now lacks. Here is a list of the IOM's recommendations and some questions that can help you relate their application to your own practice setting.

1   *Redesign processes of care to more effectively meet the needs of the chronically ill.* Whatever your specialty, you care for both individuals and groups of patients with chronic conditions. The patients with chronic conditions consume more time and resources than your other patients, so you want to be sure that you, your care team, and your patients themselves are managing care as well as possible. If you are part of a large healthcare system or belong to an IPA or Physician Association, process redesign may already be part of a larger organizational agenda into which your practice fits. If you are a private practitioner, redesign of processes of care is your responsibility. You have an opportunity to work smarter, not harder.

2   *Make efficient use of information technology* to automate clinical information and make access to that information easier for both patients and the care team. If you routinely collect demographic information about your patients and document the care that you provide, you have a head start in addressing quality of care. The important question is how well you can access the information that you have and use it along with information that is available from other sources to help you provide quality care.

   Do you spend a lot of time looking for medical records that are piled high on someone's desk? Do you have a secure website? If the answer is yes, can and do you use it interactively to allow patients to communicate with your practice? If you have already purchased Electronic Health Records (EHR) or are thinking about introducing this application into your practice, are you focusing on ways in which the technology can help you better meet the needs of your patients and your care team or are you fretting about the price? Do your practice management system, your website, your EHR, and your e-prescribing application interface with each other so you have comprehensive information from all of these sources available at your fingertips? Are you aware of the Voluntary Consensus Standards for Ambulatory Care endorsed by the National Quality Forum in the summer of 2005? Can you readily measure the quality of the care that you and your practice deliver for both individual patients and for your practice as a whole?

3   *Manage your own and your workforce's knowledge base and skills.* Your medical school and subsequent training gave you a good knowledge base, but it didn't teach you enough to sustain you for the rest of your medical career. The base of knowledge continuously expands, so even the smartest physician can benefit from the availability of new information on diagnoses and treatment. In the future, maintaining board certification and state licensure will require a commitment to life-long learning and periodic self-assessment. The same high level of competency holds true for your clinical and administrative staff. Can each one of you access information on new findings, new treatments, new medications, new administrative requirements, new administrative solutions, and most importantly, on your patients themselves?

4   *Coordinate care across patient conditions, services, settings, and time.* If you are a primary care physician or medical specialist, the office visit is the way in which you interact most frequently with patients. If you are a surgeon or hospital-based physician, your main interaction with your patients may be in a hospital or ambulatory surgery center setting, with briefer interactions in your office. Are you able to coordinate care for your patients across settings, regardless of the time of

day or night that the patients or your medical colleagues contact you? Problems with handoffs and the management of transitions from one provider to another are major sources of medical error.

5 *Enhance the effectiveness of teams.* Although the physician/patient interaction is of the utmost importance, your patients interact with other people in your office and/or at the hospital. Does everybody who interacts with patients work as a team, or do they work as individuals with little coordination of efforts? Communication skills are critical, and there is a growing awareness of the need to understand cultural, language, and literacy issues in relating to patients.

6 *Improve performance by incorporating care processes and outcomes measurement into your daily work.* Do you understand, analyze, and improve the processes that affect patient care? Do you measure the impact of what you do, set goals, and take steps to improve? Does your practice have an ongoing plan to systematically improve care?

Appendix H, which can be found on the website www.radcliffe-oxford.com/medical practicemanagement, contains a glossary of terms that are commonly used in talking about quality and quality improvement.

Examples of National Healthcare Quality and Quality Improvement Programs

Quality of healthcare and quality improvement are not new subjects. You may be familiar with and/or participate in some of the programs that already exist. Many of the current initiatives are external to medical practices and feature financial incentives for quality improvement. Although each initiative listed here has contributed in some way toward better understanding of quality problems and ways to address them, many of the externally driven programs don't affect your structure and processes for delivering care. Only you can do that.

The following list includes: disease management, centers of excellence, evidence-based medicine, practice guidelines, National Committee for Quality Assurance (NCQA) HEDIS standards, Bridges to Excellence, the Leapfrog Group, and Pay-for-Performance.

◗ *Disease management:* a systematic and comprehensive approach to improving the management of a condition.[7] The goal is to coordinate care and control costs by integrating components across the entire delivery system and by applying tools that are appropriate for the target population. One limitation of most disease management programs is that they focus on cost reduction and target the most severely ill patients. Patients do not always have a say in whether or not they can participate. Another shortcoming with disease management can be the exclusion of the primary care physician from the loop of care unless involvement of him/her is deliberately made part of the program. Although most disease management programs are not usually categorized as quality or quality improvement programs, there have been some successful efforts to improve the quality of care for chronic diseases using the Wagner Chronic Care Model and quality improvement (www.aamc.org/newsroom/pressrel/2005/050428.htm).

◗ *Centers of excellence:* the underlying premise is that there is a high correlation between volume and positive outcomes. Both the Centers for Medicare and Medicaid Services (CMS) and many managed care plans have established standards for centers of excellence.

These centers receive a single bundled fee for all services related to specific complex procedures. As with disease management, the major focus is on cost reduction, and patients do not always have input on whether or not they can seek care from a center of excellence. Again, these programs are not usually labeled as quality or QI programs, although some of them have achieved good results.

- *Evidence-based medicine (EBM):* the concept of using research evidence to make decisions about the care of individual patients has existed since the 1950s and 1960s. Since that time, the standards for evidence have become more rigorous, and the tools for assembling evidence have become more powerful and widely available.[8] Historically, one concern in using evidence-based medicine to improve the quality of care has been practicality. When information is widely scattered, busy independent physicians who are not researchers are unlikely to take the time to frame a research question, review available evidence, and select the best evidence as a guide in patient care. In order to address this issue, both the United Kingdom and the United States have made progress in synthesizing available evidence. The Cochrane Collaboration in England and the Agency for Healthcare Research and Quality's Evidence-Based Practice Centers have facilitated the organization of evidence-based medicine so that the results are easier to use. Another concern with EBM is that for a large part of medical care there is not yet solid evidence.

- *Practice guidelines:* the IOM defines clinical practice guidelines as "systematically developed statements to assist practitioner and patient decisions about appropriate healthcare for specific clinical circumstances."[7] The guidelines take evidence and move a step ahead; they build conclusions or recommendations about appropriate and necessary care for specific types of patients.[3] A problem with practice guidelines is that they depend on evidence, not all of which is reliable. A partnership of the Agency for Healthcare Research and Quality, the American Medical Association, and the American Association of Health Plans has created a National Guideline Clearinghouse that offers online access to a large and growing resource. But guidelines alone don't produce quality, particularly if there is no opportunity for physician judgment and patient feedback in their application. The real issue is that physicians do not know how to improve in a systematic and measurable way. Dissemination of evidence-based guidelines alone has not significantly changed practice performance.

- *National Committee for Quality Assurance (NCQA):* this organization sets standards for health plans and makes available comparative quality data. Its Health Plan Employer Data and Information Set (HEDIS) indicators focus primarily on the occurrence of desired or undesired events in specific population groups. Some HEDIS measures such as rates of childhood immunization and mammography deal with illness prevention. Other measures, such as the percentage of diabetics who have had an annual eye exam, focus on caring for people who have been diagnosed with a chronic illness. Similar to practice guidelines, quality measures or indicators alone do not have a major impact unless physicians know how to improve in a systematic and measurable way.

- *The Leapfrog Group (www.leapfroggroup.org):* this purchasing group was established in 2000 in order to drive "leaps" in quality and safety in hospitals by leveraging performance transparency at the provider level, consumer incentives, and provider rewards.[9] The Group includes 150 public and private purchasers and represents more than 34 million lives. Hospital participation is voluntary, and almost half of the 3000 eligible institutions have chosen to be included. Leapfrog sponsors 15 initiatives throughout the country, and its website contains the results. In a recent editorial, Dr Robert Galvin from General Electric, one of the founders of the Leapfrog Group, acknowledged that the initiative has not had the desired effect of significantly improving hospital safety.[10]

▶ *Pay-for-Performance (P4P):* Pay-for-performance programs offer financial incentives to physicians for achieving specific, measurable patient safety, quality, satisfaction, or efficiency objectives. These programs generally base a portion of physician payment on quantitative measures that may include patient care process measures, outcomes measures, or patient satisfaction scores.[11] Although pay-for-performance programs are relatively new, the programs in California and in Boston have already paid out financial rewards to physicians. Both the Medical Group Management Association (MGMA) and the American Medical Association (AMA) have developed specific standards to be met by any such programs.[11,12]

▶ *Bridges to Excellence (BTE) (www.bridgestoexcellence.org):* Spearheaded by General Electric and six other large employers, and physician leaders, Bridges to Excellence (BTE) is a pay-for-performance program that rewards physicians for delivering high quality care to patients with diabetes (Diabetes Care Link), and coronary disease (Cardiac Care Link). There is also a financial reward for the use of office-based EHR (Physician Office Link). In the diabetes and cardiac care programs, both of which are administered by the National Committee on Quality Assurance (NCQA), physicians can receive certification by meeting process and outcome goals developed by the American Diabetes Association and the American Heart Association. Because BTE uses process and outcome measures, it avoids the problem of small sample size that can penalize practices. The number of patients required for certification in each of these three programs is 35. Right now, a major shortcoming of BTE is its availability only to physicians who provide care to the patients of participating employers. BTE is considering licensing the product so that large health plans can use it.[10]

▶ *Examples of quality in office-based settings:* Organizations that have taken a leading role in promoting quality and quality improvement in office-based settings are the Institute for Healthcare Improvement (IHI), the American Academy of Family Practice (AAFP), and the American Academy of Pediatrics (AAP). Their respective websites contain the details.

Importance of Measurement in the Quality of Medicine

If measurement is the key to understanding your current status and the improvements that you make, what do you measure? The Centers for Medicare & Medicaid Services (CMS) have been working with the American Medical Association's Physician Consortium for Performance Improvement and the National Committee for Quality Assurance to measure the improvement of care for such clinical conditions as coronary artery disease and heart failure, diabetes, high blood pressure, osteoarthritis, asthma, behavioral health, prenatal care, and preventive care. In January 2005, the Performance Measurement Workgroup proposed a starter set of measures based on their ability to meet five criteria:

▶ Clinical importance and scientific validity
▶ Feasibility

- Relevance to physician performance
- Consumer relevance
- Purchaser relevance.

After an expedited review process, the National Quality Forum endorsed National Voluntary Consensus Standards for Ambulatory Care. These standards represent the consensus of more than 260 healthcare providers, consumer groups, professional associations, purchasers, federal agencies, and research and quality improvement organizations. They are a standardized set of measures for gauging and publicly reporting the quality of ambulatory care. These approved measures are available online (www.qualityforum.org) and physicians can use them voluntarily.

Public and Private Initiatives in Quality of Care and Quality Improvement

The quality of healthcare as a national concern and priority is fairly recent. Following the occurrence and publicity around numerous errors and devastating consequences, the Institute of Medicine published its 1999 report, *To Err is Human: Building a Safer Health System.*[13] That report was a wake-up call to the entire healthcare industry, and quality of care and quality improvement are now both high priorities at the national, state, and local levels. Appendix H, available on the website www.radcliffe-oxford.com/medicalpracticemanagement, lists many national public and private agencies, organizations, and associations that are concerned with both quality and quality improvement in healthcare. Check to see what is going on in your own state and local community.

Suggestions for Moving Ahead

Quality is a huge topic, and it is tempting to set it aside for another day. Rather than procrastinate about the inevitable, learn more about existing quality improvement initiatives. Use your research to gain a broad perspective so you can designate someone within your practice to organize your efforts, but remember that quality is everyone's responsibility. Then objectively assess your current situation, organize your findings, and decide what actions to take. Last but not least, document your quality efforts.

It is essential to distinguish quality improvement efforts that originate within your practice from activities that you undertake in order to satisfy external standards. Both are important. Standards that are imposed by outside agencies and organizations are likely to impact your bottom line more than the way in which you deliver patient care. If you look only outside your practice and not at what is going on within it, you won't change the structures and processes that affect your clinical results.

Learn More about Quality and Quality Improvement

So much information on quality and quality improvement is available that the challenge is in knowing where to begin. A good starting place is the Institute of Medicine's *Crossing the Quality Chasm.*[4] Although the book is long and detailed, it will give you an excellent framework, providing insights into what is wrong and how to fix it. The observations and recommendations are well documented, and you'll have the confidence of knowing that the material comes from a reliable source.

Other good places to begin your quality journey are the Dartmouth Microsystems website (www.clinicalmicrosystem.org) and *The Improvement Guide: A Practical Approach to Enhancing Organizational Performance*, by Langley *et al.*[14] The American Health Quality Association (AHQA) website (www.ahqa.org) contains both good information and links to other organizations and projects. AHQA's bi-monthly Quality Update summarizes the many quality activities and events occurring throughout the country, and its website has good information on patient safety. The Institute for Healthcare Improvement website (www.ihi.org) also has excellent information. Improvingchroniccare.org can also give you suggestions.

Quality and quality improvement are becoming an important component of the training, continuing education, and credentialing for healthcare professionals. Both the American Board of Medical Specialties and state licensure boards require physician competency in quality improvement and use of data to demonstrate that they can measure and improve the quality of care. Look at the American Board of Internal Medicine's new charter on professionalism (www.abim.org) to learn how that organization describes the quality imperative. The American Academy of Pediatrics (www.aap.org), the American Academy of Family Physicians (www.aafp.org), and the American College of Physicians (www. acponline.org) have been extremely proactive about quality, and their respective websites contain information that you might want to use in your practice. For example, the American Academy of Pediatrics EQIPP tool offers physicians assistance in managing patients with ADHD, asthma, and other conditions. The American Academy of Family Physicians Quality Initiative includes criteria for performance measures and a practice enhancement program.

The American College of Surgeons (www.facs.org) offers four programs directed toward quality improvement. These are the National Surgical Quality Improvement Program (ACS NSQIP) and accreditation of bariatric surgery, trauma, and cancer centers.[15]

If you would like to participate in training or continuing education that focuses on quality and quality improvement, investigate the programs offered by the American College of Physician Executives (www.acpe.org) and by the Institute for Healthcare Improvement (www.ihi.org). Both of these organizations have trained thousands of physicians, and their curricula are a good combination of theory and practice. Your own specialty society may also offer training.

Many of the organizations and associations that are referenced in this section hold regular meetings for which you can get CME credit. If you attend a meeting that is not limited to your specialty, you'll gain broad exposure to quality efforts throughout the country and/or state and enhance your ability to network with a wide variety of colleagues.

Designate Someone in Your Practice to be Responsible for Quality and Quality Improvement

Select one physician within your practice as the leader for your quality and quality improvement efforts. He/she will take a lead role in understanding the state-of-the-art, obtaining standards that are relevant for your practice, and in guiding your entire team to work with those standards to make systematic process improvement.

Take an Objective Look at Your Practice

A common lament from physicians is: "My practice is a mess. I need an operational audit to help me learn what is wrong and to guide me in correcting the problems." The operational audit that so many of you mention has at least three components: analysis of structure, workflow, and outcomes. Let's look at each one.

With respect to structure, two common problems have a definite impact on quality of care. One is the lack of a competent practice administrator or manager and the second is ambiguous physician responsibility for practice management. If you are one of those who say with a perfectly straight face that you "sort of have a practice manager," you indeed have a problem – and it's not your practice manager. If you "love seeing patients, hate practice management, and rotate the physician in charge so that nobody has to spend too much time doing the terrible job of managing the practice," you also have a problem. Both of these common structural problems produce the same result: your practice doesn't know what management entails, what steps you need to take, and who is responsible for each task. If you adjust and improve your structure, you'll have a better chance of improving your processes and outcomes.

Workflow process is a second issue, and it's a big one. Many of you haven't changed the way you run your practices in 30 or 40 years. If you introduce EHR into your practice before you improve your workflow, you'll automate these bad habits, not fix them. Ask yourself about the processes that are currently in place for every aspect of your practice, including but not limited to appointment scheduling, check-in, collection of demographic information, review of systems, moving the patient into and out of the exam room, prescriptions (ordering and refill), check-out, ordering ancillary tests and routing the results to physicians and patients themselves, and billing and collections. Does every process that you now have contribute positively to the delivery of care to your patients in the way in which you would like it to do?

If your workflow analysis identifies many problems, measure them, correct them, and measure them again to see how you have changed. Here are some examples. How many patients did your practice turn away because you couldn't book a convenient appointment? How many claims denials did you receive because information was incomplete and/or inaccurate? How many more patients could you have seen each day if you weren't saddled with administrative work that could have been done by someone else or electronically? Would your nurse have treated more patients if she had been able to communicate with health plans and pharmacies electronically rather than by phone? How much money did you lose because you filed claims late? How much money do your patients and insurance companies owe you?

Finally, what about outcomes? Can you do a diagnostic test on your practice to see if you can improve a quality gap? Here are practical suggestions.

▶ Explore reliable national registries to which you can submit information on your patients and from which you can receive comparative information. For example, in January 2006 Medicare implemented its Physician Voluntary Reporting Program enabling physicians to voluntarily report information on 36 evidence-based measures to the Centers for Medicare & Medicaid Services (CMS).

▶ Select a nationally accepted quality measure and apply it to 20 consecutive patients to see how good a job you are doing. There are excellent evidence-based measures available for diabetes, asthma, congestive heart failure, and preventive care.

▶ Given the structure and workflow of your practice, extract useful information about the patients for whom you care from your practice management, electronic health records, and other systems. Organize the information to tell you about patients as individuals and about subsets of patients. Do you know patients' ages and where they live? If you are a primary care physician, do you know how many of your patients have chronic conditions such as asthma, diabetes, or heart disease? For these chronic patients, do you keep careful track of important measurements, medications, and other indicators? If you are a specialist physician, do you know your most common diagnoses or procedures? If you do, are you sure that the care that you and your partners provide to this group(s) of patients meets the standards that your specialty society promulgates? Do you know how to use evidence-based medicine at the point of care?

▶ Use satisfaction surveys for patients and medical colleagues to better understand their perception of the care you provide and the processes by which you deliver it. Correct problems that you identify and check to make sure that your quality improvement activities have a positive impact on measurable results.

Organize Your Findings

If you have done a thorough job at looking at your practice, you are likely to find many areas that need improvement. Make a list of issues and organize it in a way that makes sense to you. Here's an example from a pediatric practice that had a long and overwhelming list of structural and workflow issues. The practice considered the implications of each problem. Some issues had a direct impact on patient care (e.g., communications between front office and clinicians). Other issues had financial implications for the practice (e.g., absence of revenue cycle management process). Still others were related to compliance. Clearly, the practice couldn't address everything at once. Rather than work only on enhancing financial performance or improving patient care, it selected several issues from each category, first addressing those it could easily fix. With a well-organized work plan, the practice watched its list of tasks shrink. Clinical Microsystems (www.clinicalmicrosystem.org) has a step-by-step template that takes you through a meaningful process improvement effort.

Document Your Quality Efforts

Quality improvement should be an ongoing activity in your practice. Document exactly what you do so you can determine progress and self-correct your improvement processes as you continue to learn. Documentation will also help you with accountability – to yourself, to your practice, to professional organizations, to public and private payers, and to your patients.

References

1 Brennan TA. Physicians' Professional Responsibility to Improve the Quality of Care. *Academic Medicine*. 2002; **77**(10): 973–80.

2 Audet MD, Doty MM, Shamasdin J *et al*. Measure, Learn, and Improve: Physicians' Involvement in Quality Improvement. *Health Affairs*. 2005; May/June **24**(3): 843–853.

3 Lohr KN, editor. *Medicare: A Strategy for Quality Assurance*. Washington, DC: National Academy Press; 1990.

4   Institute of Medicine. *Crossing the Quality Chasm. A New Health System for the 21st Century*. Committee of Quality of Health Care in America. Washington, DC: National Academy Press; 2001.

5   Donabedian A. *Explorations in Quality Assessment and Monitoring, Volume 1: The Definition of Quality and Approaches to Its Assessment*. Ann Arbor, MI: Health Administration Press; 1980.

6   Speroff T, O'Connor G. Study Designs for PDSA Quality Improvement Research. *Quality Management in Health Care*. 2004; **13**(1): 17–32.

7   Davidoff F. In the Teeth of Evidence. The Curious Case of Evidence-Based Medicine. *The Mount Sinai Journal of Medicine*. 1999; 66(2): 75–83.

8   Field M, Lohr KN, editors. Institute of Medicine. *Guidelines for Clinical Practice: From Development to Use*. Washington, DC: National Academy Press; 1992.

9   Galvin RS. *The US Experience with Contracting and Incentives for Quality and Efficiency: Follow the Money*. Fairfield, CT: General Electric; 2004.

10   Galvin RS, Delbanco S, Milstein A *et al*. Has the Leapfrog Group Had an Impact on the Health Care Market? *Health Affairs*. 2005; **24**(1): 228–33.

11   Medical Group Management Association. *Position Paper: Principles for Pay-for-Performance Programs and Recommendations for Medical Group Practices*. Englewood, CO: MGMA. February 2005.

12   American Medical Association. *Principles for Pay-for-Performance Programs*. March 2005.

13   Kohn LT, Corrigan JM, Donaldson MS, editors. Institute of Medicine. *To Err Is Human: Building a Safer Health System*. Washington, DC: National Academy Press; 2000.

14   Langley GI, Nolan KM, Nolan TW *et al. The Improvement Guide. A Practical Approach to Enhancing Organizational Performance*. San Francisco: Jossey-Bass Business and Management Series; 1996.

15   Petty CS. American College of Surgeons Public Information Officer, Email communications, June 8, 2005.

12 Using Information Technology to Enhance the Quality of Care, Operational Efficiency, and Revenue in Your Practice

Information technology (IT) can impact your practice in three important ways. First, it can help you improve the quality of care by reducing errors, monitoring chronic conditions, and allowing patients to become more involved in their own care. Second, it can improve the efficiency of your practice operations by streamlining processes and communications. You have more time for direct patient care if you are not searching for patient records and trying to locate other providers so you can communicate with them. Third, once you recover the cost of your investments, IT can enhance your bottom line, help you reduce your accounts receivable, and provide you with the documentation that you need to participate in pay-for-performance and other incentive programs.

The potential benefits of IT for your practice may sound too good to be true, and in fact there are caveats. Just because you introduce IT applications into your practice doesn't guarantee positive clinical, operational, and financial results. Hastily selecting vendors and products without understanding your unique needs, illogical decision-making, poorly planned implementation processes, and inattention to both staff training and managing change can have a negative impact on your outcomes. Purchasing new information technology applications without addressing office system redesign is a major mistake.

This chapter addresses the following questions:

- What are the important information technology applications for your practice?
- What are the challenges in planning and implementing information technology to support your practice?
- What questions should you ask before you contact vendors?
- What steps should you take and in what order?
- What are the keys to the successful implementation of all information technology applications?
- What can you learn from the experiences of other practices?
- What resources can help you with information technology?

What are the Important Information Technology Applications for Your Practice?

At least four information technology applications are important for your medical practice: practice management system (PMS), electronic health records (EHR), electronic prescribing (e-prescribing), and a functional website that enables you to communicate with patients and physicians. Depending on your specialty, you may have IT needs beyond these basic four.

Most practices already have a PMS that handles appointment scheduling, billing, and collection. The database contains patient demographic and financial information, including insurance coverage. When new patients come to your practice, you add their information into the existing database. After each service that you provide (e.g., office visit, procedure, consultation), you code what you have done so your PMS can generate a claim for a third party payer or for the patient. Unless you are one of the few practices still filing paper claims and unless the patient is self-pay, the claim is sent electronically to either a payer or to a clearinghouse that then forwards it to a payer. When claims are paid, you post them into your PMS. Likewise, if claims are pended for more information or denied, that information, too, goes into your PMS. You can then use the information that has been collected from various sources to run financial reports, focusing on your entire practice, individual physicians, individual patients, and/or specific third party payers.

Historically, most PMS products performed the same basic functions. They enabled you to collect demographic and financial information and extract it from the database. If you knew what information would help you manage your practice, you could retrieve it and use it in an appropriate way. If, however, you were not quite sure how to use the information in your PMS, the software didn't provide guidance. It remained an untapped reservoir.

Newer PMS systems do more than collect demographic and financial information that you later retrieve. They cross over into the realm of practice management, particularly revenue cycle management. For example, your PMS may include a code-checking feature that prevents you from filing an incomplete or improperly coded claim. One of the PMS/ revenue cycle management products that is highly ranked by national independent rating organizations does even more. The software includes the rules for submitting claims to most of the major managed care plans so you don't have to wait for denials to understand plan requirements. This product functions like a live practice manager by sorting tasks and triaging them to the appropriate staff members within your practice. For example, if your front desk schedules an appointment with a new patient, the system sends an electronic message to the person who is responsible for sending out new information packages, reminding him/her to follow through. A PMS that works like a live practice manager can completely change your workflow!

A second important application of information technology in your medical practice is the electronic health record (EHR). EHRs capture clinical information on your patients. You enter that information by using a hand-held device, voice recognition, or tablet. Some EHRs have patient portals that allow patients themselves to enter information. The EHR becomes your practice's reservoir of clinical information. You can access information related to a particular patient and/or to groups of patients. For example, if you are a family practice physician who treats many diabetic patients, you can isolate information on this group of patients in order to monitor test results and provide disease-specific patient education.

As with PMS, the technology of EHRs is evolving. Exhibit 12.4 later in this chapter describes that evolution. Right now, most EHRs are owned by a single organization such as your medical practice. Eventually, ownership may be shared by multiple healthcare organizations such as medical practices, hospitals, and other providers and services. Judging from the activities in several innovative states, there may also be information sharing through Regional Health Information Organizations (RHIOs). Looking into the future, patients themselves may own what will be called an electronic patient record (EPR). An important development for both PMS and EHR applications is the creation of integrated systems where both applications operate off the same database. If the two applications are integrated, you don't have to pay for the interface at the time of installation and on an ongoing basis when either vendor upgrades its software.

The third important IT application is e-prescribing. The percentage of patients that leave their physician's office with one or more prescriptions is high. The 2006 rollout of the Medicare part D drug benefit program provided an additional incentive for physicians to manage prescriptions as efficiently as possible. E-prescribing generally has three components. It offers clinical decision support by providing reminders and alerts and by promoting compliance with guidelines and formularies. It integrates patient data from an EHR that includes medical conditions, current and prior medications, drug allergies, laboratory results, and physician personal preferences. Combining this information can improve documentation and enhance clinical decision support. E-prescribing also facilitates communications among clinicians, pharmacies, and health plans so that these parties can transmit prescriptions, check eligibility and benefits, exchange messages, and process requests for renewal. Patients as well as clinicians can benefit from e-prescribing by saving money on the medications that they purchase.

The fourth important IT application is a website that enables you to communicate with patients and referring physicians. If you use your website for interactive communications, it can become a second portal to your practice. For example, your website can enable you to collect information on patients prior to their visit. It can allow patients to request appointments and prescription renewals, obtain test results, and pay bills online. You can communicate with referring physicians through a special website feature. If you are comfortable with the concept of virtual office visits, you can use your website to respond to inquiries from existing patients who use a credit card to pre-pay for your advice. If you do use your website for patient care, you of course reserve the right to ask your patient to come into your office for a visit.

What are the Challenges in Planning and Implementing Information Technology to Support Your Practice?

Before you contact vendors about upgrading and/or purchasing one or more of the above IT applications, take time to consider some of the planning and implementation challenges.

First, think about the future of medical decision-making. Regardless of your excellent performance in medical school, residency, and fellowship training and how much clinical experience you already have, you don't know everything. Every day brings new medical knowledge. You'll bring far more value to patient care if you know how to access information on a real-time basis than you will if you rely on what you learned and read yesterday. IT has great potential to help you enhance your clinical skills.

Second, remember that IT offers tools, not solutions. Start with your practice, not with the tools. Make sure you understand your current workflow. Do you know which processes work well and which need improvement? If not, find out. When you eventually identify vendors and products, you'll want them to address your needs. Don't make the common mistake of buying what the vendors tell you that you must have.

Third, the success or failure of IT applications is related to change. Early adopters and innovators are the exception. Most people fear change, and for good reasons. They are not sure if they can learn to do things in new ways, and they are nervous that IT tools will replace them. They won't embrace new IT applications unless you acknowledge and address these valid concerns.

Fourth, treat IT decisions as cyclical. Today's decisions may not be valid in three years. The state of the art changes, as does the corporate status of the vendors. Monitor and re-evaluate your systems regularly. If you decide to make a change in the future, your second decision doesn't necessarily mean that your first decision was a mistake. Circumstances change, and so should you.

The fifth challenge in planning and implementing IT is making a significant and appropriate financial commitment. Be careful in your evaluation of different options so you don't overspend. Why purchase a Cadillac if you only need a compact car? Exhibit 12.1 describes the experience of White Ice Internal Medicine, a 10-physician internal medicine/gastroenterology practice in Minneapolis.

EXHIBIT 12.1 White Ice Internal Medicine's purchase of an electronic health record system

White Ice Internal Medicine was a well-established internal medicine/gastroenterology practice located in Minneapolis. The practice used an external IT support company that advised the practice that the federal government required all practices to have EHRs. Without verifying this advice and without questioning the fact that the IT support company was also a reseller for a major vendor, the practice purchased an expensive client-site server system. The reseller, acting for the vendor, provided two days of training and left the physicians with the job of painstakingly converting paper charts to electronic form. Several months later, White Ice hired a new practice manager who realized that the practice had acted hastily and spent far more money than it should have. She also guided the physicians in creating and executing a realistic implementation plan.

Sixth, the attention you devote to educating and training your staff on IT and on managing the change process is more important than the IT applications that you select. Physicians can be particularly resistant to change, particularly to technological change. Involve them and your other staff in IT planning early in your planning process so everyone can absorb new knowledge before the transitions occur. Invest in your staff and you'll increase the likelihood of success.

The seventh challenge, like the previous one, relates to people. The process of planning and implementing IT applications is heavily dependent on people, so make sure you delegate internal responsibility to the right individuals. You'll need one or more physician champions, a committed practice administrator/manager, and understanding and support from your clinical staff. When you are considering applications that impact your front office and back office staff, include these people in your discussion and decision processes.

Finally, don't try to do everything yourself. You can save time and dollars and improve the quality of your IT decisions if you acknowledge your own inexperience in evaluating and implementing IT solutions. Seek external help at the outset of your IT planning process. A practice management consultant can determine whether or not you are HIPAA-compliant, educate you about the functionality of different IT applications, introduce you to reputable vendors, help you compare proposals, negotiate vendor contracts, and manage as much of the implementation as you would like. Unless you have experienced internal IT support, engage a second external consultant to help you correct any security gaps that you may have identified, check on requirements for wireless and T-1 Line access, maintain your electronic systems, and guide you in your vendor relationships once you have made and implemented your decisions.

What Questions Should You Ask Before You Contact Vendors?

If you have ever built a house, you know that the architect and builder start by asking you and your family about your needs and wants. The same principle holds true for the purchase of IT applications. Start with your practice, not with vendors and products. Before you visit a trade show or invite a vendor to make a presentation to your practice, take an inventory. What is your current workflow process? What IT applications are currently in place? What works well? Where do you have problems? With what organizations do you need to exchange clinical information? Once you answer these questions, you can explore the potential of IT to serve as a catalyst for change.

A second important question for your practice relates to timing. What is your time frame for the IT applications that you want to enhance and/or add? If you are contemplating adding, replacing, or upgrading more than one application, think about the appropriate sequence. Exhibit 12.2 describes the way a urology practice planned the replacement of its practice management system and the introduction of EHR into the practice. Exhibit 12.3 describes the experience of a pediatric practice that initially focused only on EHR and that eventually decided to purchase an integrated PMS, EHR, and document scanning system.

EXHIBIT 12.2 Red River Urology's timing in introducing its new PMS and EHR systems

---

The eleven owners of Red River Urology Associates created the practice five years ago by merging three smaller practices. New physicians joined the group, bringing the total number of physicians to eleven full-time and two part-time people. The physicians saw patients both in their main office and in space that they rented from other practices in five different locations. They needed access to both financial and clinical information in all six sites.

At the time of Red River's incorporation, the practice outsourced its billing and collection to an external vendor. This same company provided IT support. Over time, this decision proved to be unsatisfactory for the practice. To correct the problems, Red River decided to bring billing and collection in-house, engage an IT support company, purchase its own PMS, and introduce EHR into the practice. Each of these decisions had important implications for Red River's future viability.

A small IT task force, including one physician who was particularly interested in IT, the practice manager, the head nurse, and an external consultant assessed the practice's current workflow and held preliminary meetings with vendors that could provide one or both applications. The practice also asked an external IT support company for guidance before making decisions on the vendors. Red River eventually decided to purchase its PMS and EHR applications from different vendors, knowing that both companies would have to build and maintain an interface between them at the practice's expense. Red River made both purchases at the same time with the understanding that it would first implement PMS, stabilize the billing and collection, and then implement EHR.

EXHIBIT 12.3 Happy Pediatrics' IT planning for PMS and EHR

Happy Pediatrics had eight full-time and two part-time physicians. The practice had one main location and planned to open a satellite in a nearby suburb. It believed that EHR would greatly enhance the ability of the two locations to communicate with each other and facilitate coverage among the physicians. When Happy Pediatrics began its IT planning, the practice was very satisfied with its PMS vendor. The group had recently upgraded its PMS and was pleased with the quality of the service it received. The physicians were fearful of introducing two major changes into the practice simultaneously, and so they asked the vendors with which they met to demonstrate only their EHR systems.

After four vendor demonstrations, the practice realized that retention of their current PMS and purchase of an EHR from a different vendor would create problems they had not anticipated. The development and maintenance of an interface between the two vendors required them to pay an initial sum plus additional fees every time each vendor upgraded its software. As a primary care practice, Happy Pediatrics had a much smaller budget for IT than the urological practice described in Exhibit 12.2. The practice decided to purchase a single integrated PMS/EMR/document scanning system from the same vendor. Contrary to their initial goal of selecting and implementing EHR as quickly as possible, they decided to implement PMS first and activate the EHR feature on a gradual basis.

The third question for your practice relates to responsibility. Who within your practice will make the changes happen for you? In some cases, a physician champion assumes this responsibility. In other cases, an administrative person steps in. Still another alternative is to share responsibility. Regardless of your decision, be realistic about the amount of time required for your IT project(s). Make sure you don't overload the person(s) who assume responsibility for this additional work.

Fourth, step back from your own practice and learn about the future direction for IT in medical practices. Pay attention to national, state, and local policy issues and activities as well as to particular applications, vendors, and products. For example, if you are interested in EHR, educate yourself about federal, state, and regional initiatives regarding standards, interoperability, and technical assistance available to medical practices. Learn about the past, present, and future of the application itself so you don't purchase an application that is rapidly becoming obsolete.

For example, if you are interested in introducing EHR into your practice, you should learn about the evolution of the technology from computerized patient records (CPR) to electronic medical records (EMR) to electronic health records (EHR) and eventually to electronic patient records (EPR). Exhibit 12.4 contains this information. You should also understand the difference between client-site server and application service provider (ASP) models (Exhibit 12.5).

EXHIBIT 12.4 The evolution from CPR to EMR to EHR to EPR

EHRs capture data on the clinical status of individual patients, and they allow users to view in new ways information that has previously been stored. All EHRs have common building blocks, including but not limited to a database management system that allows data input in various ways (e.g., pen, voice-based technology, scanning of paper records), network through a local area network (LAN), Internet, or wireless system. EHRs also offer security, messaging, and storage of clinical information in a way that permits movement from one system to another. EHRs are an evolving technology. Earlier efforts in the 1970s were on CPRs, computer-based patient records. Next came electronic medical records (EMRs) that capture structured and unstructured data from paper and from disparate computerized systems. EMRs are usually maintained by a single organization, however. In comparison, EHRs can capture information from various sources. Still to come are electronic patient records (EPRs) that allow patients to enter information into their own records.[1]

EXHIBIT 12.5 Client-site server vs application service provider (ASP) options

When you evaluate EHR vendors and products, a major consideration will be your decision about a client-site server or Application Service Provider (ASP) as the place where your data resides. Don't confuse the question of where the data resides with ownership. You own the data regardless of its location, and your agreement with your vendor should clearly confirm this point.

In the client-site server model, you purchase one or more servers that reside in a secure location at your practice site. Your data resides on your server(s), and you are responsible for security and back-up. Software upgrades and system maintenance occur at your practice site. Although you can try to schedule routine maintenance during times when your practice is closed, your server may be down during business hours. IT emergencies, just like clinical emergencies, don't operate on schedule.

With the ASP model, you rent space from a third party entity that uses the Internet to distribute software and software-based services from a central data center to a large geographical area. The third party is your remote host, and it is responsible for ongoing security, maintenance, and upgrades. Your ASP provider usually maintains back-up servers in different parts of the country. If there is a problem with one server, one of the back-up systems takes over. You pay a monthly access fee, and there may be a per transaction fee for certain items (e.g., online bill payment). If you select the ASP model, you will want to have more than one Internet service provider.

Both the client-site server and ASP models have benefits and potential problems. ASPs are less expensive to your practice. You pay rent rather than purchase one or more servers that you must maintain. But ASP models depend on reliable Internet connectivity. Basic DSL and Cable broadband packages may not be sufficient, so you should invest in a partial or dedicated T1 line that includes a Service Level Agreement (SLA). Still another potential problem of ASP models is oversubscription. If too many users access the ASP at the same time, they may not all have the access that they thought they were getting. Again, an SLA is a good protection.

A fifth important question for your practice relates to process. What process will you use to evaluate your options and make a decision? Later sections of this chapter suggest a formal structured process and specific criteria that enable you to easily compare options.

Finally, how will you evaluate the results of your purchase? By carefully analyzing your current workflow, you can identify important indicators and establish baseline measurements. After you implement your solutions, re-measure your indicators. Hopefully you will see improvement. Many vendors will provide estimates of your return on investment (ROI). You can use this information to determine whether your expectations came to fruition. Two other ways to evaluate results of your IT innovations are to administer satisfaction surveys to your patients and staff before and after you introduce your new IT application. Exhibit 12.6 describes the way in which one of the most highly-rated PMS vendors in the country has integrated ROI into its product.

EXHIBIT 12.6 Vendor Q's emphasis on return on investment (ROI)

Vendor Q was founded in the 1990s. It offers a unique practice management system that focuses on revenue cycle management. Within six months, it will offer a second product, an EHR that is integrated with its PMS. Before Vendor Q makes a proposal to a medical practice, it requests historical information on payer mix, accounts receivable, collection, and billing and collection costs. Starting with this foundation, Vendor Q's proposal contains specific revenue cycle management goals that the vendor will help the practice achieve. Vendor Q's payment is incentive-based. If the practice doesn't achieve the mutually agreed-upon return on investment (ROI), the vendor is financially penalized.

What Steps Should You Take and in What Order?

If the prospect of addressing the ways in which IT can enhance your practice feels overwhelming, break it down into the twelve manageable steps listed in Exhibit 12.7.

EXHIBIT 12.7 Suggested steps for evaluating and implementing new information technology applications in your practice

---

1 Comply with the HIPAA Security Rule
2 Set goals and priorities
3 Create a task force
4 Develop a profile of your practice
5 Identify vendors and invite them to your practice
6 Develop a request for proposal
7 Compare and rank vendor responses
8 Make site visits and check references
9 Select the vendors and sign agreements
10 Develop an implementation plan
11 Evaluate the results
12 Start again.

Step 1: Comply with the HIPAA Security Rule

When the Health Insurance Portability and Accountability Act (HIPAA) became law in 1996, skeptical physicians and other covered entities pejoratively described it as "just another government regulation." They didn't really appreciate the ways in which the Privacy and Security Rules could protect their medical practices. As a result, they resisted compliance and directed their staff to do as little as possible on a very low budget. During the ten years since the law was passed, many of these HIPAA-phobic physicians have begun to enhance their IT applications. The light bulb of understanding has gone on and they have realized the importance of securing both protected health information (PHI) and electronic protected health information (EPHI). Start your IT planning by making sure you are HIPAA-compliant. Chapters 14 and 15 contain helpful information.

Step 2: Set Goals and Priorities

Once you're satisfied with your HIPAA compliance, set specific IT goals and priorities for your practice. What do you want to accomplish? What's a realistic timetable, given that you can't do everything at the same time? How much can you afford to spend? Set your expectations with input from the consultants and vendors with whom you are working. Exhibit 12.8 contains some examples.

EXHIBIT 12.8 Sample goals for information technology (IT) planning

GOAL	COMMENT
Upgrade DOS-based PMS.	▸ Review Windows-based systems. ▸ Consider both client-site server and ASP models.
Replace your current PMS vendor with a vendor that provides better service.	▸ Check references carefully. ▸ Review vendor ratings available from reliable national companies.
Terminate your agreement with external vendor that currently handles billing and collections, then purchase a new PMS.	▸ Your PMS will be a tool; concentrate on creating a complete revenue cycle management system.
Purchase both new PMS and EHR.	▸ Consider integrated applications as opposed to those that require one or more interfaces. ▸ If you decide to work with multiple vendors, plan and budget for the cost of both initial and ongoing interfaces.
Introduce a functional website into your practice as a prelude to EHR.	▸ Treat the website as a second portal to your practice. ▸ Website implementation is much easier than EHR and can prepare your practice for more complex changes.
Reassess your current IT support company.	▸ As the old saying goes, "Beware of two men and a truck."
Take 18 months to determine practice needs, assess options, consider vendors, make a decision, and implement new applications.	▸ Take your time; your IT decisions are about your future, so make them carefully.

Step 3: Create a Task Force

Although you will be evaluating vendors and products, enhancing IT in your practice is really about people and processes. Start by creating a multidisciplinary task force headed by a physician with an interest in IT. Make sure your practice administrator/manager, another clinician such as a nurse, and representatives of various parts of your office are part of the group.

As you may have already discovered when you decided who would manage your IT planning and implementation, one or more knowledgeable external consultants can facilitate the planning, implementation, and ongoing maintenance. Unless your practice has already experienced a similar process, you'll waste time and dollars that could be better spent. Most small and mid-size practices don't have internal IT support staff who can lead major change, so consider engaging an external IT support company.

Step 4: Develop a Practice Profile

Start with what you know best – your practice. Document the way in which every administrative and clinical process works. List your important relationships with other healthcare providers and services. Then identify strengths and weaknesses from the perspectives of the patients, physicians, and other staff. If you eliminate your practice profile and move right into vendor and product analysis, you risk automating processes that don't work well now. Exhibit I.1 in Appendix I contains a tool that can help you profile your practice before you embark on EHR planning. Appendix I is available on the website www.radcliffe-oxford.com/medicalpracticemanagement.

Step 5: Identify Vendors and Invite them to Your Practice

Now that you have set IT goals and priorities and analytically reviewed your current workflow, you are ready to contact vendors. You may already have met sales representatives at professional meetings and trade shows. Some may have contacted you and asked to make presentations to your practice. You may want to convene a preliminary meeting with one or two of these vendors just to familiarize yourself with a vendor presentation.

Take advantage of the numerous independent resources that are available to help you identify appropriate vendors. Consult these resources just as you might check *Consumer Reports* before you purchase a household appliance and the *Kelley Blue Book* before you purchase an automobile. Exhibit 12.9 lists resources on IT vendors and products and can also be found on the website www.radcliffe-oxford.com/medicalpracticemanagement.

EXHIBIT 12.9 Resources on IT vendors and their products

Professional Associations
▶ American Academy of Pediatrics
▶ American Academy of Family Physicians
▶ National professional association in your specialty

Independent Organizations/Associations that Provide Guidance on Selecting Vendors and Products
▶ The non-profit Chicago-based Certification Commission for Healthcare Information Technology (CCHIT) certifies ambulatory EHRs. By the fall of 2006, CCHIT had certified thirty-five products and extended the opportunity for certification to organizations with internally developed systems. CCHIT certification requires 100 per cent compliance with more than 200 criteria. Some of these criteria are broad functionality, evolution to standards-based interoperability with other systems, and security features that protect the privacy of personal health information (PHI).

▶ KLAS Enterprises (www.healthcomputing.com) conducts user surveys of the vendors and publishes annual "Best in KLAS" reports. Information is categorized for large and small-sized practices. The cost is $700 for physicians and higher for non-physicians. Vendors will share these reports for free.

- ❯ AC Consulting Group (www.acgroup.org) issues an annual report on EMR and EHR applications, practice management systems, mobile solutions, etc. The report ranks products based on functionality and market segment. A free report summary is available on the website. The full report is $129.95 for physicians and $229.95 for non-physicians.
- ❯ California HealthCare Foundation (www.chcf.org) publishes many reports to help practices select an IT vendor. Electronic Medical Records: A Buyer's Guide for Small Physician Practices, evaluates eight EMR products. Electronic Medical Records: Lessons from Small Physician Practices is also helpful. The Excel-based product evaluation tool by Forrester Research is also available. The information is free.
- ❯ Bcc: Consulting (www.hitbcc.com) and Unlimited Plus (www.unlimitedplus.com): This collaborative issues an EMR Guide for Small and Mid-Size Practices.
- ❯ ELMR.com contains information on more than 70 products, a vendor-feature comparison matrix, brief descriptions, a discussion forum, purchasing information, and links to vendor websites. The information is free.

Invite some of these vendors to visit your practice and make presentations. Let them know that you are at a preliminary phase of your planning process. Request general information on the company and its products that will help you understand the current and future philosophy. Develop a Request for Information (RFI) to guide the vendors, and remind them that you will ask some but not all vendors to submit a detailed proposal at a later date. Exhibit 12.10 contains topics for your RFI.

EXHIBIT 12.10 Topics for Request for Information (RFI)

- ❯ Company name
- ❯ History and future plans
- ❯ Products available
- ❯ Overview of system architecture
- ❯ Reporting capabilities and production (especially for PMS and EHR)
- ❯ Unique features (e.g., for EHR, link with data registries that are easy to use)
- ❯ Experience in your specialty and geographic area
- ❯ Approach to installation, training, and ongoing support
- ❯ General pricing

Step 6: Develop a Request for Proposal (RFP)

The vendor responses to your RFI will give you enough information to determine which vendors can potentially meet your needs. Give these vendors a formal Request for Proposal (RFP) and a deadline for submission. Exhibit I.2 in Appendix I contains sample topics for your RFP. To simplify your review, ask each vendor to prepare a cover letter that summarizes the highlights. Exhibit I.3 in Appendix I contains a sample cover letter from Best Vendor. Appendix I can be found on the website www.radcliffe-oxford.com/medicalpracticemanagement.

Step 7: Compare and Rank the Vendors

After you have obtained proposals from up to six vendors, compare their responses on the topics listed in your RFP. Scrutinize the information that you receive, since vendors use different formats. Pay careful attention to the cost information and remember to calculate your internal costs. Exhibit 12.11 contains the cost portion of a proposal from a vendor that offers an integrated PMS, EHR, and document management system. Exhibit 12.12 provides suggestions for estimating internal costs.

EXHIBIT 12.11 Vendor cost proposal for EHR

Proposal assumptions

▶ 10 full-time equivalent (FTE) users, including 2 part-time FTE physicians

▶ 1 main location and 1 satellite office

Proposal #1: ASP PMS & EMR & Document Management (Version 9.0)

▶ 3-year agreement

▶ No additional cost for future upgrades/versions of the product

▶ $5,000 ($500 x 10 providers) per month for all three applications, including PMS, EMR and Document Management. Additional users can be added at $500/provider/month. Total annual cost with 10 providers: $5,000 x 12 = $60,000.

▶ This fee includes software licensing, future upgrades/versions of the product, software support, technical support, and help desk support during normal business hours.

▶ Connection to server: $100/provider per month. Total annual costs: $100 x 10 x 12 = $12,000.

▶ Additional support and maintenance are available for an extra charge.

▶ Vendor provides the server from its hosted facilities which includes redundancy, security, encryption, backup, server maintenance, and HIPAA compliance.

▶ $590/month for clearinghouse unlimited electronic claims including Electronic Remittance Advice (ERA). Annual cost: $590 x 12 = $7,080.

Proposal #2: Client Server (Upfront) PMS & EMR & Document Management (Version 9.0)

▶ No term to the agreement; client renews the support and maintenance contract on an annual basis.

▶ No additional cost for future upgrades/versions of the product.

▶ Software Purchase Price: $55,000 upfront. Vendor can help client arrange financing if desirable.

▶ $1,325 per month support and maintenance fee starting after installation. This fee includes future upgrades/versions of the product and software support, technical support, and help desk support during normal business hours.

▶ Additional support and maintenance are available for an extra charge.

▶ Client procures server and is responsible for redundancy, security, encryption, backup, server maintenance, and HIPAA compliance.

▶ $590/month for clearinghouse unlimited electronic claims including Electronic Remittance Advice (ERA). Annual cost: $590 x 12 = $7,080.

EXHIBIT 12.12 Estimating client internal costs for implementing integrated PMS, EHR, document management solution

The cost section of the vendor proposals addresses vendor costs, not your internal costs. Make sure you understand who within your practice will be responsible for various components of implementation, and factor in those costs too. For example, if a physician champion assumes a leadership role and will see fewer patients during the time that he/she is concentrating on your new IT application(s), lower your expectations for clinical productivity and revenue generation. If your practice administrator/manager coordinates the implementation and plays an active role in staff training, make sure other staff members help with daily operational tasks. Anticipate the need for staff training as you approach the go-live date, and build that time into your schedule.

During your evaluation of the vendor proposals, look for indicators that may predict problems. Some of the common "red flags" are vendor unwillingness to collaborate with other vendors, high prices for updates, resistance to customization, corporate instability, and a track record of non-responsive customer support. Exhibit 12.13 provides additional details on these potential problems.

EXHIBIT 12.13 Vendor red flags

Unwillingness to collaborate with other vendors	If you're making a transition from one system to another, collaboration is essential. After your purchase, if you become dissatisfied with your vendor, you'll want assurance of collaboration in transitioning to a successor vendor.
Vendor charges high prices for updates	Most vendors offer free software updates once or twice each year.
Vendor resistance to customization	Every practice has its own preferences, as do the physicians within that practice. Make sure the vendor is willing to make accommodations without an additional charge.
Corporate instability	Vendors that have recently been purchased or that have recently purchased other companies may be very focused on their internal issues and neglect client service. Once these new partners are fully integrated with each other, they may reduce support for the product that you purchased.
Unavailability of support and maintenance	Information technology, like illness, doesn't run on schedule. Make sure your vendor is available 24/7/365.
Inattention to reporting capability	Just because an IT application captures financial and/or clinical data doesn't mean you can access it easily. Make sure you can get the reports that you need for decision-making purposes.

Add objectivity to your evaluation of the vendor proposals by using a numerical rating system of 1–5 that ranges from poor (1) to excellent (5). Consider weighting the features that you rank. For example, if your practice has experienced poor vendor service in the past, you can weight that quality higher than other qualities to make sure that you don't repeat the problem. Exhibit 12.14 contains a suggested method for ranking vendors.

EXHIBIT 12.14 Ranking the vendors

FEATURE	WEIGHT	#1	#2	#3	#4	#5
Functionality for your specialty	40%					
Corporate stability	10%					
Service	25%					
Cost	10%					
References	5%					
Independent ratings	10%					
All features	100%					

Step 8: Make Site Visits and Check References

After you have reviewed the vendor proposals, compared the responses, and begun to fill in your weighted rankings, you are ready to make site visits and check references. Ask the vendors for references and for the names of current clients that welcome visitors. Ask your external consultant for the names of current users that the vendor hasn't recommended so you can contact them too.

If possible, make some site visits without the vendors. Practices are more likely to be candid with you if the vendors aren't looking over their shoulders. Plan your site visits in advance so you know which members of your team will ask particular questions. Your goal is to determine how a specific product works in a specific environment. Ask the practice that you are visiting to present a clear overview of its experience with IT planning and implementation and then accompany various practice members as they use the product.

Your observations as well as the information that you learn from the practices you visit can provide valuable insights. For example, if you are evaluating EHRs, the physicians in your practice will want assurance that they can make and maintain eye contact with patients. During your site visits, watch how the physicians position the hardware. If the physician and the patient are both reading information from a screen that is conveniently placed between them, you may find them both engaged and focused in a surprisingly positive way.

Ask four key questions at the time of the site visit. First, did the vendor deliver what the client wanted on a timely basis? Second, would the client make the same decision again? Third, what went well and wrong from the client perspective? Fourth, was the vendor support efficient and effective prior to, during, and after the go-live date?

Step 9: Select the Vendor(s) and Negotiate Agreements

Now that you have your evaluations and rankings of each vendor and have obtained additional information through site visits and reference checks, you are ready to select a vendor. Narrow your list of vendors to two, not one, in order to retain negotiating leverage.

You are entering into the relationship with the best of intentions for a successful business relationship. Remember that not all relationships work out, and your agreement with the vendor is your protection. Exhibit 12.15 contains a vendor contract checklist and can be found on the website www.radcliffe-oxford.com/medicalpracticemanagement.

Read the fine print in the agreement carefully. Until you sign on the dotted line, you are still in the driver's seat. Resist vendor pressure to sign quickly. Ask an attorney who specializes in information technology to review the contract. If the vendor is new in your community, anxious to add practices in your specialty, and/or you are an influential practice, you may be able to negotiate better terms on price, length of the contract, and cost items.

Sign the agreement only after you are fully satisfied with the provisions. Then notify those vendors that you have not selected of your decision. They'll ask you why you didn't choose them, and you can tell them.

Step 10: Develop an Implementation Plan

The vendor will provide you with a standard implementation plan that lists tasks and responsibilities and lays out a timetable. Review it carefully to make sure it meets your specific needs. For example, if you prefer to phase the implementation of a particular application rather than change everything at once, make sure your vendor knows that. Also, if you have purchased different applications from different vendors, make sure that you, the two vendors, and your external IT support company collaborate to create a customized master plan. An off-the-shelf implementation plan from one of the vendors won't suffice.

Internally, take at least six important steps to facilitate smooth implementation.

- First, set a positive tone. If the IT Task Force that has made the recommendation for your practice expresses enthusiasm, it can set the tone for the entire practice.

- Second, acknowledge that change raises people's anxiety levels. Ask your clinical and administrative staff about their concerns rather than pretend that they don't exist. Once people voice their worries, you can address them so they don't become barriers to success.

- Third, clearly describe the goal, steps, and timetable. Everyone in your practice will appreciate good communication at the outset and throughout the transition process.

- Fourth, recognize that people learn in different ways and at different paces. Some people are visual learners, and others prefer to read instructions. Ask the vendor(s) to make multiple methods of learning available. These might include "webinars", in-person tutorials, online assistance, and printed quick guides.

- Fifth, rely on your practice and not the vendor(s) for training. Even though you have paid for training as part of your purchase, you know the people in your practice better than the vendor. Identify your own super-users and coaches who can help others in the practice. Nobody can learn everything at a single training session, so make sure to make training available on an ongoing basis.

- Sixth, be realistic about the bumps and surprises that will occur along the way regardless of how carefully you, your consultants, and the vendors have planned the transition. You won't see improvements in efficiency and productivity on day one, so emphasize the long-term value of the change for your practice.

Step 11: Evaluate the Results

If you asked yourself the right questions at the start of your IT planning and implementation process, you already know the importance of evaluating the results. Exhibit 12.16 identifies measurements that you can use to evaluate three applications, PMS, EHR, and an interactive website with the ability to communicate with patients and clinicians. This exhibit can be found on the website www.radcliffe-oxford.com/medicalpracticemanagement.

Step 12: Start Again!

Now that you have evaluated your needs, assessed your options, made one or more choices, implemented your solutions, and evaluated the results, you have completed the IT planning and implementation cycle. Start again. This time correct any problems that you experienced the first time around. Consider IT planning and implementation as an ongoing activity for your practice.

What are the Keys to Successful Implementation of All Information Technology Applications?

Although the preceding sections of this chapter offer many suggestions for successful implementation of IT applications, some are more important than others. Medical practices that have had positive experiences with IT applications generally mention the following keys to success:

▶ Identify a physician champion who is not only interested in introducing new IT applications, but who is able and willing to coach his or her peers through the transition process. This champion should be willing to test the new application(s) on his own patients, work with one or more vendors, and then train medical colleagues and other staff.

▶ Enlist the commitment of all physicians in the practice, including those who are comfortable with the new applications and those who are not.

▶ Plan the timing to suit your practice. There's no right way to innovate. Some practices choose a massive conversion, while others prefer gradual change. The decision is up to you.

▶ Pay close attention to the relationships between multiple vendors and support companies. You selected the vendors and the products, so you are in charge. You understand your practice better than any vendor, so retain control of training and transition.

▶ Purchase the level of support that is appropriate for your practice. If you are a mid- to large-size practice and your internal staff can handle major projects, delegate the work to them. If your practice is small and you are skeptical about the capability of your internal staff to take on new and complicated projects, engage one or more external consultants.

What Can You Learn from the Experiences of Other Practices?

The positive and negative experiences of other practices can teach you more about decision-making processes than they can about vendors and products. Exhibit 12.17 describes the experiences of two practices. The first practice took one year to plan the implementation of an EHR system to interface with its existing PMS. That practice had a very positive experience with the change. The second practice made a hasty decision to purchase EHR and wrote about the debacle in the *Annals of Internal Medicine*.

EXHIBIT 12.17 Two practices' experience with the introduction of EHR into the practice

Florence Family Medicine had 13 full-time physicians and 45 other staff members in its two locations. The opening of its second location motivated the practice to investigate the replacement of its paper medical records with EHR. At the time of this important decision, the practice was satisfied with its current PMS vendor, and so it looked only at the one IT application. The practice allowed itself a full year to plan its approach, assess its needs, select a vendor, and implement its new system.

One physician and two senior administrative staff members, including the practice manager, shared responsibility for guiding the transition. From the perspective of this small and dedicated team, the transition went smoothly for several reasons. The practice did not rely on the vendor to train its people. The two senior administrative people on the EHR team coached each member of the practice on an individual basis. The training included practice sessions using both the new hardware and software. Shortly before the go-live date, the practice deliberately reduced its patient schedule to accommodate the training. By design, the entire practice went live simultaneously in order to prevent less enthusiastic members of the practice from remaining wedded to paper records. The practice also engaged its patients in the change. Rather than emphasizing the difficulty of change, it described its new EHR as a practice enhancement designed to better serve patients.

Seven years have passed since Florence Family Medicine implemented its EHR system. In retrospect, the only thing that the practice regrets is that it didn't purchase extra hardware at the outset. As it learned over time, when hardware breaks or wears out, as it always does, it's wise to have spare equipment on hand.

By contrast, Greenhouse Internists in the Philadelphia area had an extremely negative experience with its EMR implementation. In 2005, the four physicians in this practice wrote a candid and discouraging article in the *Annals of Internal Medicine*[2] describing the problems. In the practice's own words, "We were forced rapidly to adjust our work flows during implementation, which seemed akin to redesigning an airplane in flight . . . Going live rendered everyone in the office incompetent to do their core jobs." Greenhouse did not take time to assess its needs, to talk with multiple vendors, and to plan its implementation. It rushed the purchase and the implementation. Although none of the physicians would return to paper records, the experience could have been much more positive for the practice.

What Resources Can Help You Learn More about Information Technology?

Take advantage of the many available resources on IT support for medical practices. Exhibit 12.9 earlier in this chapter listed resources for identifying vendors that might meet your needs. Exhibit 12.18 lists organizations that focus on IT, magazines and trade journals, physician practice management organizations, physician professional organizations and societies, and books and articles. This exhibit can be found on the website www.radcliffe-oxford.com/medicalpracticemanagement.

References

1 Satinsky MA. Electronic Medical Records and the Development of Electronic Health Records and Electronic Patient Records. *North Carolina Medical Board Forum*. 2004; **3**: 4–9.

2 Baron RJ, Fabens EL, Schiffman M *et al*. Electronic Health Records: Just around the Corner? Or over the Cliff? *Annals of Internal Medicine*. 2005; **143**(3): 222–6.

13 Corporate Compliance

Although the topic of corporate compliance generates more disinterest and outright disdain than other aspects of medical practice management, it is essential to the business of medicine. Like it or not, managing your current services and/or adding new ones without a good understanding of the relevant federal and state laws and regulations is risky business. Here's a good parallel in your personal life. Supposing you purchased a lot, built a house, and made numerous additions without checking the relevant licensing requirements and building codes? You would expose yourself to numerous penalties for violating the law. Your medical practice is no different.

This chapter was developed with the assistance of Steven M Shaber and Wilson Heyman of Poyner & Spruill, LLP, Raleigh, NC. It addresses the following questions:

- What is corporate compliance and why do you need a corporate compliance plan?

- What aspects of your practice should you target in developing a corporate compliance plan?

- What laws and regulations affect corporate compliance, and what are the penalties?

- What steps should you take to develop a corporate compliance plan and to implement and maintain a corporate compliance program?

- Other than healthcare corporate compliance, what are some of the other laws and regulations with which your practice should comply?

What is Corporate Compliance and Why Do You Need a Corporate Compliance Plan?

A corporate compliance program is "the collection of internal mechanisms or steps that an organization implements to prevent and detect violations of law." It includes documentation of the program, procedures, responsibilities, and activities that must be implemented and continuously maintained for the plan to be deemed effective by the authority that can potentially sentence those in violation.[1] An important concept in corporate compliance is what, if anything, the individual or organization did prior to any investigation. If an investigation determines that there was a serious attempt to address compliance, this finding may lessen blame and punishment.

Although the concept of corporate compliance is important in healthcare, it isn't unique to the field. In fact, corporate compliance is an outgrowth of government concerns in the 1980s about improprieties in the defense industry. The industry itself created the Defense

Industry Initiative in order to set standards of conduct, develop self-policing, encourage ethical business conduct, develop public accountability, and encourage compliance.[2] Also, the Sentencing Reform Act of 1984 (28 USC 994) established Federal Sentencing Guidelines to standardize and increase the predictability of federal court sentences.[1] The Guidelines encouraged organizations to be proactive and to put in place internal mechanisms for prevention, detection, and reporting of potentially criminal conduct. Such mechanisms can reduce criminal penalties for misconduct, provided that they are actually followed.

As a physician in medical practice, you need to know what laws and regulations affect the way in which you do business. If either the government or individuals are successful in proving that your practice was out of compliance with relevant laws and regulations, there are civil and criminal penalties. Although these penalties can be stiff, keep in mind that compliance programs are *voluntary*, unless your practice is operating under a corporate integrity agreement that has resulted from a previous violation of Medicare law. You don't have to take every step that is recommended in this chapter, but there's great value to your practice if you do.

There are at least four advantages of developing a corporate compliance plan for your practice:[1,3]

▶ *Risk reduction:* An active corporate compliance plan can reduce the likelihood that you'll violate the law. If you violate the law, an active program may reduce your penalties. A sham program, however, can increase penalties.

▶ *Most effective use of legal counsel:* Corporate compliance is technical and complicated. Good advice from legal counsel is essential. If you have a formal corporate compliance plan, you can appropriately engage outside legal counsel to ensure that your documentation and communication procedures maximize the use of attorney/client privilege. Another advantage of having a plan is that legal counsel knows what you are doing and can respond rapidly if needed.

▶ *Employee training:* A compliance plan provides you with a means to train your employees on the appropriate handling of search warrants, unannounced searches, and other aspects of compliance. You need buy-in from your workforce for a compliance plan to reduce your risk and to help you respond to investigations.

▶ *Communicating changes:* A corporate compliance plan is your blueprint for compliance. When you want to make changes in policy or incorporate new legal requirements, you can do it easily if you already have protocols in place.

What Aspects of Your Practice Should You Target in Developing a Corporate Compliance Plan?

Although corporate compliance affects your entire practice, there are specific aspects of running a medical practice that subject you to greater risk. In 2000, the Office of Inspector General (OIG) in the US Department of Health and Human Services (HHS) identified some of the most common risks.[4] These are listed in Exhibit 13.1 which can also be found on the website www.radcliffe-oxford.com/medicalpracticemanagement.

EXHIBIT 13.1 Common risk areas for physician practices

POTENTIAL RISK	COMMON EXAMPLES
Coding and billing	▶ Billing for services you didn't provide ▶ Billing for supplies and equipment you didn't use or that weren't reasonable and necessary ▶ Duplicate billing for a service that results in excess payment, or billing for a service for which another payer has reimbursed you ▶ Billing for non-covered services ▶ Using the provider number of a physician other than yourself ▶ Failing to comply with the "incident to" billing requirements for the services provided by nurse practitioners and others ▶ Failing to comply with requirements for physician supervision of non-physicians ▶ Failing to use appropriate modifiers in your coding ▶ Clustering (i.e., using one or two codes consistently under the assumption that they will average out) ▶ Unbundling services that must be coded and billed as one ▶ Billing for a higher level of service than you actually provided (i.e., upcoding) ▶ Failing to comply with the requirements for contracting with third party billing companies
Reasonable and necessary services	▶ Submitting to Medicare claims for services that are not considered reasonable and necessary in cases other than when you need the denial to submit the claim to another payer
Medical record documentation	You must meet standards for: ▶ Completeness and accuracy ▶ Reason for the encounter, relevant history, findings during the exam, prior diagnostic test results, diagnosis, care plan, date and identity of observer, rationale for ordering diagnostic and ancillary testing, identification of health risk factors, patient progress, responses to treatment, and changes in diagnosis
Completion of CMS-1500 form	You must: ▶ Link CPT and ICD-9 codes with the reason for the visit/service ▶ Use appropriate modifiers, provide complete information about a beneficiary's other insurance coverage.
Improper inducements, kickbacks, and self-referrals	▶ This provision applies to arrangements between your practice and outside entities. Examples are joint ventures, consulting contracts, medical directorships, office and equipment leases, and gifts and gratuities.
Retention of medical and business records	Make sure you have: ▶ Policies and procedures on record retention (medical and business) that comply with federal and state requirements ▶ Documentation of investigations of potential compliance violations.
Other	▶ Physician compliance with Patient Anti-Dumping statute ▶ Arrangements for professional courtesy

Source: *Office of Inspector General*[4] and *Johnson*.[2]

What Laws and Regulations Affect Corporate Compliance and What Are the Penalties?

A good corporate compliance program helps prevent you from violating both federal and state laws governing corporate compliance. Given the variability in state statutes, this section identifies only the relevant federal statutes. Be sure to ask counsel about state statutes that may apply.

▶ *False Claims Act (FCA):* This law has existed since the Civil War. Changes in 1986 have made it more effective. This is the law that is most frequently used to prosecute healthcare providers, and the relevant provisions are those dealing with fraud against the Medicare and Medicaid programs and against the federal government. The FCA "prohibits knowingly submitting a false or fraudulent claim for payment or approval" to Medicare, Medicaid, or another federal healthcare program.[2] *Knowingly* means a practice deliberately submitted a claim it knew to be false, deliberately remained ignorant of requirements by not keeping up-to-date on changes in laws and regulations, and/or recklessly disregarded the law. The potential civil penalty for violation of the FCA is between $5,000 and $10,000 for each false claim plus treble damages on the false claims subject to certain exceptions.

▶ *Civil Monetary Penalties Act:* This law prohibits providers from submitting claims that he/she *knew* or *should have known* weren't medically necessary, were furnished by an unlicensed or unsupervised physician, were furnished by a physician who obtained a license to practice by misrepresentation, were provided by a physician who was not a participant in that particular federal health program, or who offered a monetary or other inducement to the beneficiary as an inducement to use that provider. The monetary penalty can be as high as $10,000 per item/service, and as with the FCA, treble damages apply.

▶ *Stark Self-Referral Prohibitions:* The Stark law applies to physicians (but not mid-level providers such as nurse practitioners and physician assistants) who refer Medicare and Medicaid patients for specific services, called "designated health services" (DHS), to entities with which they or an immediate family member have a financial relationship, unless there is an exception under the law or in implementing regulations. Stark applies to what goes on within physician practices as well as to financial relationships between physicians and organizations outside the practice to which the physicians refer such patients.

   Although the list of DHS is prescribed by the Stark law, the Center for Medicare and Medicaid Services (CMS) by rule interprets that list to define services that qualify as designated health services (DHS). Because this interpretation changes, be sure to check the current information on the CMS website (www.cms.hhs.gov/medicare/currentcodes.pdf). DHS includes the following:

   — Clinical laboratory services

   — Physical therapy, occupational therapy, and speech and language pathology services

   — Radiology and certain other imaging services such as MRIs

   — Radiation therapy services and supplies

   — Durable medical equipment and supplies

   — Parenteral and enteral nutrients, equipment, and supplies

— Prosthetics, orthotics, and prosthetic devices and supplies

— Home health services

— Outpatient prescription drugs

— Inpatient and outpatient hospital services.

The Stark law is highly technical, and in general, violations have three characteristics:

1 There is a financial relationship between a physician (or a physician's immediate family member) and an entity that provides a DHS;

2 There is a referral of a Medicare or Medicaid patient by the physician to that entity for the purpose of furnishing a DHS; and

3 None of the exceptions excludes the arrangement from the statutory prohibition.

The parties' lack of intention to violate the law is not a protection.

Stark prohibits the individual or entity that receives a prohibited referral from billing Medicare or Medicaid, the patient, or any third party. Any payment that is received in violation of the law must be refunded, and Medicare or Medicaid will deny payment for any such services. Violations of the Stark statute can also result in a $15,000 civil monetary penalty for the physician that makes the improper referral and for the individual or entity that files the claim. There can also be a civil monetary penalty of $100,000 for circumvention schemes. Physicians and entities that are found to be in violation of Stark can be excluded from participating in Medicare and Medicaid.

So what are the exceptions to the Stark law? Exceptions that apply to individual physicians include:

— Properly designed and documented space and equipment leases

— Bona fide employment relationships

— Properly designed and documented personal service contracts

— Certain physician incentive plans in the managed care setting

— Remuneration unrelated to the provision of designated health services

— Properly designed and documented hospital and physician recruitment contracts

— Physician payments to laboratories or other entities for ancillary services

— Isolated transactions involving the one-time sale of property or a practice

— Certain arrangement contracts between hospitals and group practices for services billed by the hospital

— Certain properly designed and documented fair market value compensation arrangements for the provision of physician services

— Certain indirect compensation arrangements.

For physicians who practice in a group practice, as defined by Stark, there is also an in-office ancillary services exception that has very technical and specific requirements. Some of these requirements relate to operating as a bona fide group practice, the range of patient care provided by group members through the practice, the compensation system, and the relationship of the compensation system to the volume or value of DHS referrals.

In order to determine whether or not the Stark statute applies to an arrangement that you are considering, begin with three important questions. First, does the arrangement involve referral of a Medicare or Medicaid patient by a physician? Referral is defined somewhat broadly and includes a physician request for service/item/good payable under Part B, a request for a consultation and all the services that are ordered as a result of the consultation, and a prescription for a course of treatment. Referrals also apply to referrals among colleagues within a physician group. Second, is the referral for a designated health service? The third question applies to exceptions to the Stark statue. Many though not all of these exceptions require that compensation be made at "fair market value" as compared with other prices for the same services in the community agreed to in an arm's length transaction. Many of the Stark exceptions also require that compensation be calculated in a way that does not take into account the volume or value of referrals.[4]

One of the most commonly asked questions about Stark is whether or not it applies to the referral of your own patients to your own nurses or technicians for ancillary services that you perform in your office. Provided you qualify as a group practice and meet standards regarding who provides the service, where the service is provided, and what billing number is used, you can make these referrals. Be cautious, however, and regularly check the OIG's Advisory Opinions. The landscape can change.[5] Another commonly asked question relates to referrals from one physician to another in the same group practice. The regulations allow this type of referral to a physician who is a contracted physician in the group without requiring that the physician be a member of the group as an owner, employee, or locum physician. There are also requirements for both supervision and productivity bonuses.

▶ *Anti-Kickback Act of 1986:* Many physicians confuse the Stark statute with the anti-kickback statute. They are not the same, as shown in Exhibit 13.2 below.[5,7] The Anti-Kickback Act of 1986 prohibits the offer, payment, solicitation, or receipt of remuneration that is even partially in return for:

1 The referral of patients (or arrangement for referral) to others for the provision of items or services for which payment may be made under any federal healthcare program

2 The purchase, lease, or order (or arrangement for such) of any good, facility, service, or item for which payment may be made under any federal healthcare program.

Thus, the Anti-Kickback statute applies to referrals of any item or services reimbursed under a federal healthcare program by *any* party, not only by physicians, if some additional value is exchanged.

EXHIBIT 13.2 Differences between Stark and Anti-Kickback statutes

ISSUE	STARK	ANTI-KICKBACK
Application to healthcare professionals	Physicians, including chiropractors and dentists, but not mid-level providers.	Anyone engaging in business with a federal healthcare program.
Intent	Bad intent not required.	Specific intent required.

(continued)

ISSUE	STARK	ANTI-KICKBACK
Boundaries	Defines boundaries of permissible behavior. The only way to overcome the prohibition in the statute is to explicitly comply with an exception.	Describes transactions that may tend to induce referrals but don't necessarily violate the law. Even if transactions don't meet a safe harbor, they don't necessarily violate the statute.
Penalties	Civil monetary penalties.	Exclusion from federal healthcare programs, criminal penalties of up to $25,000 in fines and/or up to 5 years in jail, and $50,000 civil monetary penalty/violation.
Relationship of the statutes	Although Stark applies to a more limited set of healthcare providers and services than anti-kickback, if it applies, it applies regardless of your intentions. Make sure to analyze every situation under both statutes.	The safe harbors to anti-kickback and the exceptions to Stark are not identical. Make sure to analyze every situation under both statutes.

Source: Gosfield, AG.[5,7] www.aafp.org/fpm.

The penalty for violating the anti-kickback statute is a felony criminal offense punishable by up to 5 years' imprisonment and/or a $25,000 fine. All parties to the transaction may be sanctioned. In addition to the criminal sanctions, there are civil sanctions, including monetary penalties and exclusion from all federal healthcare programs. The tax-exempt status of a hospital or other exempt facility can be jeopardized by violation of the statute.

The anti-kickback statute is so broad that it is often difficult to determine the legality of transactions and relationships between healthcare providers and entities. In order to provide guidance, the Office of Inspector General (OIG) in the Department of Health and Human Services (HHS) has issued regulations that describe *safe harbors*, advisory opinions, and fraud alerts. Exhibit 13.3 contains examples of safe harbors that may relate to physician practices. Although the OIG is helpful, its guidance is not definitive. An arrangement that does not meet the requirement of a safe harbor may not be illegal, and the only way to find out is to test the arrangement in a court of law. What really counts is intention to induce referrals, but the government is allowed to "prove" your intentions by inference (i.e., by pointing out the reasonable implications of your actions).

EXHIBIT 13.3 Safe harbors for physician practices

The following transactions come within the safe harbors, provided they are properly put together and documented:
- Certain investment interests
- Certain arrangements involving the rental of space and equipment
- Certain personal service and management contracts
- Bona fide employment arrangements
- Certain transactions involving the sale of physician practices
- Warranties and discount arrangements
- Referral services

❱ Transactions involving group purchasing organizations

❱ Waivers of beneficiary co-payments and deductibles

❱ Certain price reductions offered by providers to health plans

❱ Practitioner recruitment arrangements

❱ Obstetrical malpractice insurance subsidies

❱ Investments in group practices

❱ Investments in ambulatory surgical centers

❱ Referral arrangements for specialty services

❱ Hospital and large group subsidies for physician acquisition of Electronic Health Record (EHR) and e-prescribing systems provided the subsidies are used for software, IT, and training services and that physicians pay at least 15 percent of the cost.

Sources: Johnson, B.[2] and Terry, K.[8]

❱ *Exclusion:* In addition to the financial damages and penalties described in the preceding sections, physicians can be excluded from federal health programs such as Medicare if they violate laws governing these programs. Various felony convictions lead to mandatory exclusion. Other criminal or civil violations lead to permissive exclusion at the discretion of the government.

What Steps Should You Take to Develop a Corporate Compliance Plan and Implement and Maintain a Corporate Compliance Program?

Once you make the commitment to develop a corporate compliance plan, here are the steps that you should take.

❱ *Involve legal counsel:* Involve your attorney from the outset so you can take advantage of the attorney–client privilege and work–product rules. If the attorney who assists you with other aspects of your practice is not well-versed in corporate compliance, request a referral to someone else in the same firm or in another firm who has the expertise that you need.

❱ *Review available information:* Although your attorney will provide guidance for you, take advantage of the excellent information on compliance that is available from the federal government. Be sure to review the US Federal Sentencing Guidelines including the seven minimum steps for a compliance program. The OIG's Compliance Program Guidelines for Individual and Small Group Physician Practices, OIG model compliance plans, and the annual OIG Compliance Workplan are also good resources. The OIG is particularly sensitive to differences in practice size and resources that make large and expensive compliance efforts unrealistic in many situations. Exhibit 13.4 lists these and other good resources on corporate compliance and can be found on the website www. radcliffe-oxford.com/medicalpracticemanagement.

❱ *Obtain formal written endorsement for the development of a corporate compliance plan from your practice's governing body:* Buy-in and support from the ownership of your practice is essential. Formal endorsement of your intention to go forward with corporate compliance sends a message to your entire workforce as well as to any law enforcement personnel who may become involved. In developing your practice's formal endorsement of corporate compliance, make sure to mention the specific legal counsel that you have engaged to help you. Be clear about the time when attorney–client privilege begins.

▶ *Decide if you will develop your compliance plan internally or purchase outside assistance:* Keeping in mind the internal resources that you have to devote to corporate compliance, decide whether you will ask a member of your workforce to do the bulk of the work or if you will engage external consulting assistance. If you decide to engage an outside consultant, make sure that you hire someone who is willing to teach you the details. After you develop and implement your initial corporate compliance plan, evaluate it on an annual basis. Make sure you know how to do this work.

▶ *Develop a position description for your compliance officer and designate an individual to assume responsibility:* The development, implementation, and regular review of your compliance plan require oversight. First prepare a job description and then decide who will do the job. Most practices with ten or fewer physicians designate one or more people within the practice to assume this responsibility.

▶ *Develop a code of ethics for your practice that asserts your commitment to corporate compliance:* Your code of ethics reaffirms your commitment to corporate compliance and serves as the basis for a statement of support that every member of your workforce should sign.

▶ *Do a risk assessment for your practice:* Once you know the requirements for corporate compliance, identify areas for which you may be at risk. At this point in the compliance process, you are looking at broad topics, not specific details. Here's an example. Medicare and Medicaid have many coding and billing requirements. If you know that your practice is not up-to-date on these requirements and that you don't perform a regular coding audit, coding and billing is an area of risk for you. As you move to the next steps on this list of tasks, you can identify the details.

▶ *Create an implementation team:* Involve your outside legal counsel, your compliance officer, and other members of your practice in your investigation of your current compliance efforts. Make sure all these people as well as other members of your workforce understand that all conversations are confidential.

▶ *Conduct a baseline audit:* After you complete your risk assessment, you are ready to move onto a baseline audit in all the important areas of corporate compliance. You know which areas are of risk, and you can devote particular attention to them. Conduct the audit by reviewing the systems and documents that are currently in place. Interviews with employees and with outside agents with which you deal are other important sources of information. Do not overlook the fact that if you wish, this audit can be done under the direction of counsel so it is covered by the privilege and work–product rules.

▶ *Revise position descriptions:* Your baseline audit will provide you with detailed information on those aspects of your practice that present potential compliance risks. At this point, many practices realize that their risks exist because responsibilities within the practice are unclear. You may want to revise position descriptions.

▶ *Review and modify operating policies and procedures:* Your baseline audit may also show that operating policies and procedures don't address compliance issues. Now is the time to make appropriate changes.

▶ *Review and modify personnel policies and procedures:* Your baseline audit may show that your personnel policies and procedures need revision. For example, many practices realize that they have not asked their workforce members to sign written statements in support of corporate compliance and that they do not have appropriate disciplinary procedures.

▶ *Develop internal audit processes:* Your initial compliance audit is just the beginning of a process that should be ongoing. The goal of compliance is to detect and correct any problems on an ongoing basis. You need an internal audit process that helps you meet this goal.

▶ *Establish internal communications and reporting systems:* Compliance doesn't mean perfection; it means you can detect and fix problems, and then follow up those actions by communicating what you have done throughout your workforce and to any outside agents with which you deal. Make sure you have systems for spreading the word as appropriate.

▶ *Report back to the governing body:* After you complete your risk assessment and audit and make necessary changes in your job descriptions, operating policies and procedures, personnel policies and procedures, internal audit processes, and internal communications and reporting systems, complete the cycle by reporting back to the governing body of your practice that formalized corporate compliance in your practice.

▶ *Educate and train your workforce:* Educate and train your workforce. Follow-up on your initial training with regular refresher training.

▶ *Evaluate and modify the compliance plan on an annual basis:* Use your initial corporate compliance plan as a starting point. Each year, evaluate and modify your plan so that it is always up-to-date.

Other than Corporate Compliance, What Are the Other Major Areas of Compliance with Which You Should Be Concerned?

Your practice should comply with federal and state laws and regulations beyond healthcare corporate compliance. For example, you must comply with the requirements of the Occupational Safety and Health Act of 1970 (OSHA). If you provide laboratory services within your practice, you must comply with the requirements of the Clinical Laboratory Improvement Amendments (CLIA). Compliance with the Health Insurance Portability and Accountability Act (HIPAA) is covered in Chapters 14 and 15.

References

1   Aspen Health Law Center, Aspen Reference Group. Corporate Compliance Programs for Group Practices. In: *Medical Group Practice: Legal and Administrative Guide.* Gaithersburg, MD: Aspen Publishers; 1999–2003. 13i–13:57.

2   Johnson BA. Corporate Compliance in a Medical Practice Setting. In: Thomas MS and Keagy BA, editors. *Essentials of Physician Practice Management.* San Francisco: John Wiley & Sons; 2004.

3   Willging P. Corporate Compliance Isn't Just 'More Government'. www. nursinghomesmagazine.com, January, 2004, pages 18–21.

4   Office of Inspector General, Notice, "Compliance Program for Individual and Small Group Physician Practices," *Federal Register*, October 5, 2000, **65**(194), 59434–52.

5   Gosfield AG. The Stark Truth about the Stark Law: Part I. *Family Practice Management*. 2003; **November/December**, 2003: 27–32.

6   Johnson BA. Reading the tea leaves. Making sense of new legal guidance on ancillary services. *MGMA Connexion*, 5, 6 July 2005.

7   Gosfield AG. The Stark Truth About the Stark Law: Part II. *Family Practice Management*, **February**, 2004: 41–45.

8   Terry K. Feds to hospitals: It's okay to help docs get IT. www.memag.com. August 18, 2006.

14 An Overview of HIPAA Compliance

The Health Insurance Portability and Accountability Act of 1996 (HIPAA) has been called the most important piece of healthcare legislation since Medicare and Medicaid. The Act gave the federal government the ability to mandate the ways in which healthcare plans, providers, and clearinghouses store and transmit individuals' personal healthcare information. Until the passage of HIPAA, no national or industry standards governed the privacy and security of an individual's health information.

HIPAA has four parts, the Privacy Rule, the Security Rule, Transactions and Code Sets Standards, and National Identifiers. This chapter focuses on the Privacy Rule and the Security Rule, the two parts of the Act which fall into the Administrative Simplification category and which require significant process changes in medical practices that meet the federal definition of covered entities. This chapter addresses the following questions. Read it in conjunction with Chapter 15 and Appendices J and K on the website www.radcliffe-oxford.com/medicalpracticemanagement:

- Who must comply with HIPAA?
- What is the purpose and history of HIPAA, and how can it benefit your practice?
- What is the timetable for implementing all four parts of HIPAA?
- How does the government enforce compliance with the HIPAA Privacy and Security Rules?
- What are the similarities and differences between the HIPAA Privacy and Security Rules?
- Who should be your practice's Privacy and Security Officials?
- What steps should you take and in what order to comply with the Privacy and Security Rules?
- What factors are likely to contribute to successful compliance with the Privacy and Security Rules?

Who Must Comply with HIPAA?

HIPAA applies to covered entities such as health plans, healthcare clearinghouses such as billing services, and any healthcare providers (e.g., physicians, hospitals, nursing homes) that transmit health information in electronic form in connection with a HIPAA transaction. If you are a medical practice and/or an employer that offers health insurance to your employees, you should comply with the requirements.

What Is the Purpose and History of HIPAA, and How Can It Benefit Your Practice?

The Health Insurance Portability and Accountability Act of 1996 addressed two major problems in healthcare. One of those problems was the portability of health insurance. Historically, employees who changed jobs could not take their health insurance with them. As job changes have become more prevalent in our society, the portability dilemma has affected more members of the workforce. The portability section of HIPAA permits employees to continue their health insurance without waiting periods or pre-existing condition restrictions under certain circumstances. HIPAA also addressed the need to standardize the transmission of certain administrative and financial information and to simultaneously protect the privacy and security of personal health information.

Since the passage of HIPAA in 1996, the federal government's rolling timetable for implementation of each of the four sections of the Act has required practices to develop and implement new and different approaches for protecting personal health information. Even before the passage of HIPAA, compliance was not a popular topic with physicians. The intense focus on HIPAA compliance has caused many practices to ignore the important benefits that HIPAA can bring to them. These benefits include but are not limited to:

▸ Improved accuracy and efficiency in posting accounts receivable

▸ Automatic posting of payments to your bank account

▸ Automated insurance eligibility checks that tell you who has insurance coverage and the amount of the co-payments and deductibles

▸ Streamlined claims filing process that can accelerate reimbursement

▸ Reduction in the time that clinical staff spend on administrative processes so they can devote more time to patient care

▸ Building a strong and secure foundation for information technology applications that can enhance your quality of care, operational efficiency, and financial management.

What Is the Timetable for Implementing All Four Parts of HIPAA?

In developing and implementing HIPAA, the federal government followed its standard process. First, it wrote the Act, dividing it into four components. For each component it issued proposed regulations for implementation and for soliciting public comment prior to issuing final rules. Based on the input it received from both organizations and individuals, the Department of Health and Human Services (DHHS) published a final rule that included two dates, the date on which the rule became effective and the compliance date.

Exhibit 14.1 shows the HIPAA timetable for all four parts of the Act.

EXHIBIT 14.1 HIPAA timetable

COMPONENT	FINAL RULE PUBLICATION	COMPLIANCE DATE*
Transaction and Code Set Standards	08/17/00	10/16/02 (no extension) or 10/16/03 (with extension)
Privacy Standards 2003	12/28/00	04/14/03

(continued)

COMPONENT	FINAL RULE PUBLICATION	COMPLIANCE DATE*
Security Standards	04/21/03	04/20/05
National Identifier Standards	05/31/02 – employers 01/23/04 – providers	07/30/04 – employers 05/23/07 – providers
*Small health plans with less than $5 million in revenue have an additional year to comply.		

Source: Department of Health and Human Services (DHHS)

How Does the Government Enforce Compliance with the HIPAA Privacy and Security Rules?

Although HIPAA was passed in 1996, the government did not publish an Enforcement Rule until April 18, 2005. It is still too soon to know if this Rule will signify the start of a new enforcement era. Nonetheless, HIPAA contains standards that you should treat as requirements. If you have postponed starting on HIPAA Privacy and Security Rule activities because the burden of compliance feels overwhelming, rethink your position. If your practice is a covered entity under HIPAA, failure to voluntarily comply puts you at risk for both civil and criminal penalties. Furthermore, it puts you at risk for very negative publicity about your practice.

The DHHS has designated the Office of Civil Rights (OCR) to be responsible for implementing HIPAA. The OCR has the right to:

▶ Investigate complaints received from individuals and organizations that believe that a covered entity such as your medical practice is not complying with the HIPAA Privacy and/or Security Rule standards

▶ Assist covered entities in achieving voluntary compliance with the Privacy and Security Rules by providing technical assistance

▶ Make determinations regarding exemptions to the preemption of state law (applies primarily to the Privacy Rule).

During the years between the compliance dates for the Privacy and Security Rules and the issuance of the Enforcement Rule in 2005, the government was not proactive in enforcing either Rule. It focused on providing technical assistance to facilitate voluntary compliance. The OCR did not schedule regular site visits to medical practices and other covered entities to audit compliance. Rather, if and when individuals or organizations filed complaints within 180 days of an alleged occurrence, the OCR responded to the complaint and, if appropriate, investigated the practice. In situations where there was an investigation, the practice was required to comply with the OCR's request to provide documentation of HIPAA compliance activities. Improper use or disclosure of either protected health information (PHI) or electronic protected health information (EPHI) could result in both civil and criminal penalties, including fines and imprisonment.

Between the compliance date of April 14, 2003 and May 31, 2005, the OCR received more than 13,000 complaints under the Privacy Rule. It did not levy any civil monetary penalties, but it did refer 200 cases to the Department of Justice for potential criminal action. There was one criminal conviction case in Seattle, where a hospital worker stole patient information for use in identity theft (www.hhs.gov/ocr/hipaa).

What Are the Similarities and Differences Between the HIPAA Privacy and Security Rules?

The Privacy and Security Rules complement each other. The Privacy Rule protects personal health information (PHI), and the Security Rule protects a subset of PHI, electronic protected health information (EPHI). Examples of EPHI are electronic data transactions, email communications, practice management systems, personal digital assistants, text pagers, and website portals. Paper-to-paper faxes are not considered to be EPHI, but computer-generated faxes are. Voice telephone communications are not considered to be EPHI, but computer-based voice response units are.

Although there are similarities in the implementation of both the Privacy and Security Rules, there are also differences. Medical practices that have implemented both Rules have taken similar steps to compare their current practices with standards and to identify gaps between the existing situation and government expectations. For both Rules, this gap analysis becomes the foundation for taking corrective action, documenting your actions, regularly training your staff, and monitoring compliance on an ongoing basis. Both Rules require written policies and procedures, Business Associate Agreements, adherence to a "minimum necessary" need-to-know policy, employee sanctions for breach, designated responsibility, and preventive safeguards.

Although the processes for implementing the two Rules have similarities, for many practices, the differences between them have made the implementation of the Security Rule the more challenging. These differences are: breadth of coverage, degree of direction, allowable management discretion, and division of responsibilities for implementation.

Breadth of Coverage

With respect to breadth of coverage, the Privacy Rule deals primarily, although not exclusively, with your practice's business operations. You can therefore satisfy the Privacy Rule requirements by designating responsibilities and by developing and implementing specific policies and procedures. The Security Rule covers not only parts of your business operations, but also administrative, physical, and technical safeguards. Security rule compliance goes well beyond designating responsibility and developing policies and procedures. Depending on what you learn about your practice during the gap and risk analysis stages in your Security Rule implementation process, you may decide to make major modifications in your physical facility and/or technical data security.

Degree of Direction

With respect to direction, the Security Rule is more directive about securing EPHI than the Privacy Rule is about securing PHI. The complexity of security creates the difference. Think about the many ways in which information technology applications already do or could support your practice in the future. You might have a practice management system, electronic health records, e-prescribing, web-based interactive functions, a lab computer, and many other electronic functions.

Allowable Management Discretion

The Security Rule allows more management discretion than does the Privacy Rule in two ways. First, the Security Rule was deliberately written to acknowledge differences among practices. It is organized into *standards* and *implementation specifications*. The standards contain broad issues that all practices should address, and the implementation specifications support those standards. Implementation specifications can be *required* or *addressable*, giving you a great deal of discretion in what you do. The meaning of *required* specifications is clear; you must meet them. The meaning of *addressable* specifications can be confusing. Addressable doesn't mean optional; it means that you must review each specification and either implement it as it is written or document why you can't. If you can't implement a particular specification, you must implement another measure that in some way meets the related standard.

The Security Rule offers you more management discretion than the Privacy Rule in a second way. Rather than prescribe what you *should* do, it encourages you to determine what you *could* do and then make decisions about what is appropriate for your practice. After you have identified gaps between your practice and the standards and specifications, the likelihood of the occurrence of adverse events, and the estimated cost of fixing your problems, it is up to you to decide what, if anything, you will do and in what order. Implementation of the Security Rule thus relies on your judgment. With the Security Rule, you can't borrow a colleague's solution. Each practice is unique, and you should develop your own response.

Division of Responsibilities for Implementation

Finally, the two Rules differ with respect to responsibility for taking corrective action. With little exception, most practices have the internal ability to develop the policies and procedures that they need to comply with the Privacy Rule, provided someone within the practice takes the time to do the work. Although some practices seek guidance from an external consultant, with good direction most of them can do the bulk of the work themselves. The Security Rule is different. Not all practices have the internal expertise to perform gap and risk analyses and take corrective action. By necessity, many practices call in outside experts to help with some or all of the work. Exhibit 14.2 describes the experience of Gornish Medical Group.

EXHIBIT 14.2 Gornish Medical Group's experience with security rule compliance

---

Gornish Medical Group used three consultants in developing and implementing a Security Rule compliance program. A general practice management consultant helped the practice's multidisciplinary Security Rule Task Force establish a logical work process and complete both gap and risk analyses. Based on the findings, the practice determined that it had the internal capability to fix some but not all of the problems. For example, the practice could easily secure doors and windows (physical security). It needed help from a seasoned information technology consultant to review options for securing its on-site server. These two consultants helped the practice develop and implement its Security Rule compliance program. The practice eventually contracted with an information technology consultant to provide ongoing assistance not only with Security Rule compliance but also with other information technology-related tasks.

Who Should Be Your Practice's Privacy and Security Officials?

Compliance with both the Privacy and Security Rules requires that your practice designate one or more individuals as your Privacy and Security Rule Officials respectively. Before you make a decision, review the following four options.

▶ Option 1 is to designate the same person as both the Privacy and Security Official. As described above, the processes for implementing the two Rules have many similarities, even though the scope of the Security Rule is far broader. You may decide that one physician or your practice administrator/manager has the ability and time to assume responsibility for compliance with both Rules.

▶ Option 2 is to designate two people to share the responsibilities for both Privacy and Security. Particularly if you have nothing in place and are developing two new programs, as opposed to maintaining programs that have already been created, the responsibility is large and complex. A clinical/administrative team may work best for you.

▶ Option 3 is to designate two different people within your practice as the Privacy and Security Officials. You may find that a physician and/or practice administrator/manager are comfortable with one but not both of the Rules, so you can divide up the work.

▶ Option 4 is to engage an external consultant as your Privacy and/or Security Official, or to help you with a portion of the work. For both Rules, an external consultant can develop customized policies and procedures more quickly than you can, letting you review and modify the work. Using an external consultant to help with the Security Rule makes good sense for small and mid-size practices where staff are already handling multiple tasks and cannot set these responsibilities aside to work on large special projects. If you do engage one or more external consultants to help you with either Rule, make sure that the consultant(s) is clearly accountable to someone within your practice.

In order to decide which of the four options described above is appropriate for your practice, take the time to learn about the substance of each Rule and then review the sample job descriptions for a Privacy Rule Official and a Security Rule Official located in Appendix K on the website www.radcliffe-oxford.com/medicalpracticemanagement. Particularly when you are developing as well as implementing compliance programs, success depends on good organizational skills, leadership, and a willingness to learn new concepts.

Exhibits 14.3 and 14.4 are examples from two internal medicine practices in North Carolina. The practices are similar in size and specialty, but different in management style. Gornish Medical Group, the practice described in Exhibit 14.3, was committed to a team approach for both Rules, and it created better understanding and buy-in from the entire workforce than at Tall Oaks Internal Medicine, the practice described in Exhibit 14.4.

EXHIBIT 14.3 Gornish Medical Group's approach to HIPAA Privacy and Security Rule compliance

Gornish Medical Group has seven full-time and one part-time physicians. The total workforce, including the physicians, is 50 people. One of the physicians is Empire's Managing Partner, and the other partners take responsibility for particular projects as appropriate. The physician who is particularly interested in Privacy is the Privacy Official, and a different physician who is more interested in information technology is the Security Official. The practice manager and representatives from different parts of the office (front office, back office, nursing staff), as well as the appropriate Privacy and Security Officials worked as teams to develop and implement the appropriate steps for each Rule. Gornish also engaged external consultants to help it organize information and work processes, perform gap and risk analyses, write customized policies and procedures, and take corrective action regarding physical security and technical standards and specifications.

EXHIBIT 14.4 Tall Oaks Internal Medicine's approach to HIPAA Privacy and Security Rule compliance

Tall Oaks Internal Medicine has eleven full-time physicians. The total workforce, including the physicians, is 70 people. Tall Oaks has a practice administrator, and the partners in the practice asked him to handle compliance with both the Privacy and Security Rules. For the Privacy Rule, one physician and representatives of each part of the office formed a work group to determine what the practice would do and how it would do it. The assistant administrator and a physician assigned to the work group played a major role. For the Security Rule, however, the practice administrator handles the project himself without organizing an internal team. The practice engaged an external practice management consultant for both Rules to help it organize information and processes, perform gap and risk analyses, write customized policies and procedures, and take limited corrective action. Tall Oaks was much less aggressive than Gornish Medical Group in correcting security problems, and there was minimal knowledge and buy-in from the workforce on Security Rule issues.

What Steps Should You Take and In What Order to Comply with the Privacy and Security Rules?

Although the Privacy and Security Rules have both similarities and differences, the recommended steps for compliance with each Rule are similar. These steps are:

- Learn the basic information about the Privacy/Security Rules.

- Perform a gap analysis to determine how your practice compares with the provisions of each Rule.

- Develop and implement policies and procedures.

- Train your workforce when you implement your compliance programs and provide regular updates.

- Document your activities on an ongoing basis.

- Monitor both programs on an ongoing basis and make appropriate modifications.

Learn the Basic Information about the Privacy/Security Rules

A good rule of thumb for both the Privacy and Security Rules is to learn basic information before you take action in your practice. Chapter 15 covers the important concepts for each Rule. Appendix J contains a glossary and Appendix K contains additional sources of information on the HIPAA Privacy and Security Rules, including recommended websites. Chapter 15, and Appendices J and K can be found on the website www.radcliffe-oxford. com/medicalpracticemanagement. Once you know what you have to do, you can create a process that makes sense for you, given the size of your practice, the skills of your workforce, and your budget.

Perform a Gap Analysis to Determine How Your Practice Compares with the Provisions of Each Rule

Once you know the basics about each Rule, you are in a position to compare your current practice operations with the standards that the government has promulgated. Many of the resources that are listed in Appendix K on the website www.radcliffe-oxford.com/medicalpracticemanagement contain checklists that you can use to assess your practice. Physically walk around your practice with your checklists, inspecting your practice and comparing what you have in place with what you should or could have in place.

Many practices engage an external consultant to perform the gap analysis for the Privacy and/or the Security Rule. The advantage to using outside help is that an experienced consultant can quickly identify your gaps and suggest ways to make corrections that have worked in other medical practice settings.

For the Security Rule, you need to take one more step after you complete your gap analysis. The Security Rule has required and addressable implementation specifications, giving you the discretion to do what is appropriate for your practice. Review the additional information about the Security Rule provided in Chapter 15 on the website www.radcliffe-oxford.com/medicalpracticemanagement with respect to the Security Rule and risk assessment.

Develop and Implement Policies and Procedures

For both the Privacy and Security Rules, you must develop policies and procedures on specific topics. Appendix K on the website www.radcliffe-oxford.com/medicalpractice management lists the topics that must be addressed by each rule and provides sample policies and procedures.

Pay close attention to the format of the policies and procedures. You should specify at least the following information:
- Your practice name
- Policy name and number
- Purpose/objective
- Responsibility within your practice
- Procedure
- Forms related to your policy and procedure
- Dates originated, reviewed, and revised
- Authorized signatures.

Train Your Workforce

Workforce training on both Rules is mandatory. If you train carefully, you reduce the likelihood that workforce members will make an unintentional or intentional error. When you implement your compliance programs, provide introductory sessions for your entire workforce and then provide periodic updates on an ongoing basis. Most practices have frequent staff turnover, so don't assume that new members of your workforce are knowledgeable about this important topic. Be sure to document attendance. Some practices administer a short quiz to make sure that people understand the basic principles.

If you are comfortable with the subject matter, do the training yourself. If not, ask an external consultant to provide assistance. Everybody doesn't need to know everything, so develop training that is appropriate for your audience. For example, if you have a HIPAA Privacy and/or Security Task Force, these people need to know more details than the rest of your workforce.

Document Your Activities on an Ongoing Basis

Both the Privacy and Security Rules require that you document your activities. Your policies and procedures are an important source of written documentation about your programs. Keep good records on workforce training, complaints brought to the attention of your practice, and steps that you have taken to correct any problems. The rule of thumb here is: "When in doubt, write it down." Many practices that are computer savvy set up their compliance programs electronically so they can easily keep track of what they are doing.

Monitor Both Programs on an Ongoing Basis and Make Appropriate Modifications

After you implement your HIPAA Privacy and Security compliance programs, regularly review your written policies and procedures and the reaction of your workforce and Business Associates to what you have put in place. Make changes when and if appropriate, and be sure to document what you do.

What Factors Are Likely to Contribute to Successful Compliance with the Privacy and Security Rules?

The following factors can contribute to successful compliance with both the Privacy and Security Rules: physician commitment, managing your compliance programs in an organized and accountable manner, getting outside help when you need it, and actively involving your workforce.

Physician Commitment

Physician commitment to compliance with both the Privacy and Security Rules sets the tone for the entire practice. If you yourself understand the importance of the Rules and communicate to both clinical and non-clinical staff that compliance is mandatory, not optional, in your practice, you will motivate the entire team to do a good job.

Managing the Project in an Organized and Accountable Manner

HIPAA is complex. The concepts and requirements of both the Privacy Rule and the Security Rule may be new to you, and you'll need to take many steps to comply. Organizing your process and making sure there is clear accountability is equally as challenging as the subject matter itself. Practices that recognize and manage the complexity of developing their compliance programs are the most likely to succeed.

Getting Outside Help when You Need It

You may want to get help from one or more external consultants for two reasons – time and experience. With respect to time, the development of HIPAA Privacy and Security compliance programs is time-consuming. If you can't designate one or more competent member(s) of your workforce to assume responsibility for both projects without seriously jeopardizing your practice operations, ask an outsider for help. A consultant can do the work more efficiently and thoroughly than you can. Second, particularly with respect to the Security Rule, an experienced consultant may have the information technology/security experience to help with your gap and risk assessments and the correction of any problem areas that you identify.

As always, if you engage one or more external consultants, be clear in your directions, communicate your expectations, and clarify the ways in which your outside experts and your workforce will collaborate.

Actively Involving Your Workforce

Finally, involve members of your workforce in the development and implementation of both the Privacy and Security Rule compliance programs. Select representatives from different disciplines (e.g., physician, nurse, front desk, billing and collections, administration) to be part of your Privacy and Security Rule task forces so you get input from all parts of your office. When your task forces understand what you are doing, they'll communicate the message to other workforce members.

15 HIPAA Privacy Rule and Security Rule Concepts

The entire text of this chapter is available on the website www.radcliffe-oxford.com/medicalpracticemanagement.

Appendix A: Steps for Creating a Strong Foundation

Follow these steps in the suggested order if you are starting a new practice, moving your practice, and/or reviewing the way you have set up and manage your current practice. The abbreviations stand for: Organization and Management (OM); Financial Management (FM); Managing Staff and Outside Resources (HR); Improving Healthcare Delivery and Clinical Outcomes (DO); and Compliance (C).

1 **Determine your start-up or move date (OM):** Determine when you want to open your doors to patients and allow yourself six to nine months to put everything in place. Real estate will be a key factor in your timing. The availability of a building that you buy or space that you lease will dictate your timetable. **Make the decision on start-up or moving date with your advisory team, including your attorney, certified public accountant, banker, realtor, and practice management consultant. You must complete this task before you open or move your practice.**

2 **Obtain legal advice on the appropriate corporate structure (OM):** You have choices in the legal structure for your practice. Select an attorney with medical practice experience to help you make and execute this decision. Make sure your attorney drafts the appropriate supporting documents. Not all situations work out, so protect yourself and your associates. Complete this task before you open or move your practice and review your decision regularly. Exhibit A.1 and Exhibit A.2 describe two practices that paid little attention to corporate structure and documentation and came to regret their negligence.

EXHIBIT A.1 Eagle Surgical Associates' mistake

Dr Bald and his wife founded Eagle Surgical Associates in 2000; the Balds were co-owners of the practice. Within three years, the volume of patients had grown exponentially, and the Balds were ready to add another physician. Dr Bald knew a physician in his specialty from his military service, and he invited this surgeon to join him as a salaried employee on a part-time basis. Although the Balds had an attorney, they ignored the advice of counsel and did not draft any legal documents. A gentlemen's agreement was sufficient for them. Within three months, it became clear that the new physician was not working out. Terminating the relationship with the new physician was difficult and costly because there was no employment agreement or clarity about non-compete restrictions.

EXHIBIT A.2 Delayed dissolution of Happy Pediatrics

Happy Pediatrics had two owners. Both pediatricians had previously worked for a staff model health plan that had closed its doors. The practice employed a third pediatrician on a part-time basis. When the practice started, the partners asked the attorney husband of the salaried physician to do the incorporation, but no partnership agreement was put in place. Over time, the three pediatricians realized that they were incompatible in a private practice setting. There was a nine-month delay before the physicians could dissolve the practice and open separate practices because the initial legal work had never been completed.

3 **Decide what services you want to provide (OM):** You'll want to provide the basic services for which you are trained, and you'll have options about other revenue-producing services. You don't have to offer everything at once, and you should make your decision based on realistic financial projections. **Work with your accountant and your practice management consultant to make this decision. Make it early in your process because the services that you provide to patients will drive many other decisions that you make.**

4 **Draft or revise the fee schedule for your practice (FM):** Once you have decided on the services that you will provide, list the CPT and/or facility codes that you will use to bill for your services. Decide what fees you will charge. Many practices set their fees at an across-the-board percentage of Medicare. It's wise to develop your code and fee information as soon as possible so you can work with the various payers, particularly the managed care companies. When you apply for credentialing and network status, you can ask each payer for its reimbursement by specific code. Some but not all payers will request the fees that you actually charge, so you should have that information too. **An external consultant with experience in managed care can help you with this task.** Although some physicians don't complete this task until after their practices are open, **make every effort to do it ahead of time. Then review your fees regularly and make changes when appropriate.** Why not be reimbursed for your services at the very outset? Exhibit A.3 describes the experience of Capitol Internal Medicine.

EXHIBIT A.3 Capitol Internal Medicine's reimbursement problems

Capitol Internal Medicine was one of 11 practices formerly owned by a large community healthcare system. The arrangement had not been satisfactory to either party, and so the physicians bought their practice back. In their haste to remain in the provider networks of the managed care plan in which they were already participants, the physicians accepted whatever fee schedules the managed care plans offered them without leveraging their size and number of patients to negotiate better rates. Within a very short time, the physicians realized that they were receiving much lower rates than they had previously received. They hired a consultant to go back to each plan, provide the appropriate information, and negotiate higher fees. The renegotiation took six months because of plan-specific internal issues. Had the practice been more careful at the outset, they would have received higher reimbursement much sooner.

5 **Begin work on your practice logo and other identity pieces (OM):** When you are ready to open your doors to patients, move to a new location, promote a new service that you offer, or give your existing practice a fresh look, you will want to tell

physician colleagues and the community about your practice. The marketing world calls your logo, your stationery, and your business card your "identity piece." **Resist the temptation to save money by asking your talented children to help with this task and seek professional guidance from an external marketing consultant and/or graphic designer.** You may want to coordinate your new look with your décor. **Complete this step before you open or move your practice.**

6 **Review and decide on information technology for your practice, including but not limited to your practice management systems (PMS), an interactive website, electronic health records (EHR) system, e-prescribing, and the integration among these applications (DO):** Information technology can help you create an efficient and cost-effective practice. If you are already in practice, IT can help you improve efficiency, quality of care, and financial performance. If you are just starting out in practice, you may decide to set yourself up as a "paperless" office so you don't later have to convert from paper to electronic mode. If you are moving your practice, you may decide that the change in location is an ideal time to change your IT applications. Regardless of why IT has your attention, the sooner you know what applications and vendors will support your practice, the more quickly you can make decisions about staff, space, and layout. **Get help from an external information technology consultant, and complete this task before you open or move your practice.**

7 **Determine your requirements for location and space and select a site (OM):** Once you know what services you will provide when you open or move your practice and what services you might like to add at a later date, you can look for a location and for space that meets your needs. You yourself may know something about real estate, but remember that residential and commercial transactions are different. **Work with a real estate consultant who represents you as the tenant or purchaser.** It goes without saying that **you need to select your site and space in order to open your practice.**

8 **Obtain telephone and fax numbers, an email address, and a practice website (OM):** Before you open your doors, you'll be filling out a great deal of paperwork. If you have your contact information ahead of time, you can provide complete information. Most managed care plans won't process your application for credentialing until they have all these details. **Complete this task yourself well before you open or move your practice.**

9 **Ask your attorney to develop a Compliance Plan for your practice (C):** A compliance plan developed by your attorney will guide you in compliance with the Stark, anti-fraud and abuse, HIPAA Privacy and Security, and other government programs. **Collaborate with your attorney on compliance, and address this task before you open or move your practice.**

10 **Familiarize yourself with the requirements of the HIPAA Privacy and Security Rules (C):** HIPAA is a relatively recent aspect of compliance. The law governing it was passed in 1996. HIPAA Privacy and Security Rules protect the confidentiality of protected health information (PHI) and electronic protected health information (EPHI). As soon as you decide on your location and site and before you begin working on your interior layout, make sure you understand the HIPAA basics. If you are already in practice, HIPAA applies to you too. **A general practice management consultant with knowledge of HIPAA** can provide guidance. Later in your start-up process, after you have hired your staff, he/she can give your team more specific assistance. At this point, you need to know enough to help you make informed decisions about building and

interior design; as you get closer to the opening of your practice, you can make sure you have your policies and procedures in place and that your staff are trained. **You can do this task yourself, and you should complete it before you open or move your practice. If you are already in practice, the dates for compliance have passed, so make sure your policies and procedures are documented and implemented.**

11 **Contact/meet with an interior design firm regarding office layout and décor (C):** If you are setting up a practice or moving, you must think about the inside of your practice as well as the site and location. If you are already in practice, you should also pay attention to layout and décor. The services that you provide and the ways in which you use information technology to support your practice will affect your decisions on layout and décor. Be sure to comply with the requirements of HIPAA Privacy and Security Rules. **Consult with an interior design firm that specializes in medical practices.** If you get things right at the start, you won't have to redo them. **You need to start this task before you open or move your practice; you do not need to complete it before opening day.**

12 **Obtain/amend your state medical license (OM):** You must have a license from your state medical board to practice medicine in the state where your practice is located. Make sure you obtain or amend your license before you apply for medical staff privileges, malpractice insurance, and participation in the various managed care provider networks. **Complete this task yourself before you open or move your practice.**

13 **Obtain/amend your medical malpractice coverage (OM):** Opportunities for malpractice coverage vary by state. Ask your state Medical Society or Department of Insurance for carrier names and then comparison shop for coverage and price. Make sure you purchase the level of coverage that the payers require, and be careful about tail coverage. When you apply for credentialing with different payers, you must provide proof of coverage. **Complete this task yourself, and make sure that your coverage is in place before you open or move your practice.**

14 **Obtain your federal tax ID number (OM):** As soon as you incorporate your practice, request a federal tax ID number www.irs.gov/business/small/index.html). The managed care companies and other payers will ask you to provide it. Go to the IRS website and contact your attorney if you have questions. **Complete this task yourself before you open or move your practice.**

15 **Register your practice with the Secretary of State and other appropriate state and local agencies (OM):** You have a small business, and you'll need to register with the Secretary of State and/or other appropriate agencies in the state(s) and city(ies)/county(ies) where your practice is located. Ask your **attorney** for guidance. **Complete this task yourself before you open or move your practice.**

16 **Submit/amend application(s) for hospital privileges (OM):** If you've done your homework before you select the city/town and actual site for your office, you already know to which hospitals you want to apply for privileges. The Medical Staff office at each hospital will provide guidance. You must provide recommendations, copies of licenses and board certification, your drug enforcement administration (DEA) numbers, verification of professional liability insurance, and documentation and proof of expertise in certain procedures. The application and approval processes can take several months, so start as soon as possible. The managed care companies and some

of the other payers will not review your applications for credentialing until you have hospital privileges. **Complete this task yourself. Start far enough in advance so that you are properly credentialed at one or more hospitals before you open your practice. If you are moving your practice to a new location, make sure to give adequate advance notice to the hospitals where you have privileges. If you are a member of any hospital committees, contact them directly.**

17 **Obtain a National Provider Identification Number (FM):** A single 10-digit number that contains no intelligence about you or your practice will enable you to conduct electronic claims and other HIPAA-regulated transactions. The Centers for Medicare & Medicaid Services (CMS) has contracted with FOX Systems Inc. to act as the NPI Enumerator and handle support operations, process applications, and operate a customer service center. Obtain your NPI by contacting the NPI Enumerator by phone (800 465-3203 or 800 692-2326), by email (customerservice@npienumerator.com), or by writing to NPI Enumerator, PO Box 6059, Fargo, ND 58108-6059. **Complete this task yourself as soon as possible.**

18 **Apply to become part of the networks for one or more managed care plans or, if you are already in these networks, update your information (FM):** Most physicians become part of one or more managed care provider networks. If you aren't, you may find that patients won't come to your practice and/or medical colleagues won't refer to you.

Dealing with managed care plans is complicated since there is such variation in requirements and reimbursement. Ask your state Medical Society or colleagues in your community for the name of a reputable consultant who can do the following for you before you open or move your practice: advise you which plans are important in your community; check to see if the important plans are accepting new providers; determine the credentialing process; using the CPT and facility codes for the services and procedures that you will provide/perform, obtain the proposed reimbursement from each plan; review the contract language; and follow through on the credentialing application and contract. If you are already in practice, make sure you know what is going on with your managed care contracts or consider outsourcing the responsibility to a practice management consultant.

19 **Apply for participation in Medicare and Medicaid, or if you are already a provider, amend your information (FM):** If you are starting a practice and have no patient base, you will need to make decisions about participation in Medicare and Medicaid. Contact your Medicare intermediary and your state Medicaid agency to get information about credentialing and claims submission. Make sure you know the rules for both programs. Ask a **consultant** for assistance and complete this task **before you open or move your practice** so that you can receive reimbursement from public payers as soon as possible.

20 **Obtain/amend your federal and state narcotic licenses (OM):** You must have both federal and state licenses to prescribe narcotics. The Department of Justice Drug Enforcement Administration Form 224 is available at www.usdoj.gov/dea. **Complete this task yourself before you open or move your practice.**

21 **Select a banker and arrange for a bank loan if necessary (OM/FM):** Your banker will be important to your practice not only at the start, but also in the years to come. Talk with colleagues in the medical community to identify banks that have a private banking division. Get recommendations for particular individuals who are experienced

in dealing with medical practices. Select your banker before you complete your business plan. **Handle this task yourself, since the personal chemistry between you and your banker is something only you can determine. Complete this task before you open your practice.**

22 **Review your office lease or other documents with your attorney (OM):** By now you know whether or not you will build, purchase, or lease. Review your decision and documents with your attorney. **Complete this task yourself before you continue in the start-up or moving processes.**

23 **Prepare a list of the fixed assets that you would like to purchase (FM/DO):** When you know what services you will provide and the location(s) and site(s) of your office, list the fixed assets that you would like to purchase and get some price quotations. Make a complete list even if you ultimately decide that you won't purchase everything at one time. If you are using an interior design consultant, he/she will have good working relationships with office furniture and other companies. **You'll be spending a lot of time in your office, so make sure it is comfortable for you. Do this task yourself. After you hire a practice administrator/manager, get his/her assistance. Collaborate with an interior design consultant. Complete this task before you open or move your practice.**

24 **Prepare a strategic business plan for your practice and develop the supporting financial information (i.e., budget, operating statement, cash flow projections and balance sheet) and implementation plan (FM):** Your business plan is for you and the entire team with which you will work. It should contain your mission, vision, goals and objectives, strategies, action steps, timing and delegation of responsibilities. You'll need supporting financial information and an implementation plan. **Collaborate with an external consultant, your accountant, and your banker to prepare this document. Complete this task before you open or move your practice and make strategic business planning an ongoing part of your practice management.**

25 **Open a business checking account (FM):** Once you have selected your bank, you can open a business checking account. **Complete this task yourself before you open your practice, or if you are moving to a new location, give the bank your new contact information. Make sure to specify who in your practice will have signatory authority.** In some practices, the physicians sign all the checks. In others, the practice manager as well as one or more physicians can sign.

26 **Obtain a state(s) unemployment tax identification number (HR):** As an employer you should register with your state's Department of Employment Security. Check the IRS website for state-specific information (www.irs.gov/business/small/index.html). **Complete this task yourself before you open your practice.**

27 **Develop your employee compensation package (HR):** Your employee compensation package includes both salaries and employee benefits. A good way to learn about hourly wage and annual salary ranges for practice managers and other employees is to check with the state chapter of MGMA, the professional organization for practice administrators. With respect to the benefits, you have options about the benefits that you offer to your employees and their families. An insurance broker can give you information on health and dental insurance, short- and long-term disability insurance, and life insurance. Then decide if you want to offer tuition benefits, a retirement plan, and other benefits. You personally should decide on your wages, salaries, and benefits

before you hire employees so you can make this information part of the offer. **Review the compensation package periodically.**

28 **Develop a job description and hire a practice administrator or practice manager (HR):** You have made good progress so far, but there's a great deal left to do. If you plan to hire a practice administrator or practice manager, do it now. Make sure to develop a job description and salary range. Advertise and interview multiple candidates for the position. Be careful in your interviews and reference checks; this is one of the most important decisions you will make. Once you make your selection, you can ask for help with the remaining tasks. **Complete this task yourself before you open your practice. Throughout the life of your practice, review your decision and make sure you have the right person for the job.**

29 **Schedule implementation and training for your practice management system, web-based communications, and electronic health records (DO):** Now that you have selected your important IT systems and hired a practice administrator/ manager, you can determine when you will hire your remaining staff and schedule implementation and training for all your systems. Put these dates on your schedule well in advance of your start-up or move so that everything works smoothly when patients arrive. **You and your practice administrator/manager can jointly make the arrangements so that the implementation and training are completed and have been tested before you open or move your practice.**

30 **Clarify the requirements for Medicare and Medicaid billing (FM):** If your practice will file claims with Medicare and Medicaid, make sure you know the coding and billing requirements for each of these programs. Both your practice administrator/manager and billing supervisor should pay a personal visit to representatives of each program to make sure you are clear. **Complete this task before you open your practice and begin seeing patients. Each year, the Office of Inspector General publishes a work plan that lays out priorities. Make sure you remain current on new developments.**

31 **Test the claims submission processes for every government and private payer (FM):** You want your coding, claims submission, claims follow-up/resubmission, and collections for every payer to work without a glitch. If you are starting a practice, moving, or replacing or upgrading existing systems, plan and test every detail with every payer. Take advantage of opportunities for direct claims submission that bypass clearinghouse intervention; you'll get paid faster. If your claims do go through a clearinghouse, make sure you understand the relationship between the clearinghouse and your practice management system. **You, your practice administrator/practice manager, and your billing staff should assume responsibility for this task, and you should do it before you open your practice.**

32 **Determine your payment and collection policies (FM):** As the owner of your practice, make sure you establish clear payment and collection policies. Even if your practice management system automatically invoices payers and individuals and/or you use a collections agency, you are the decision-maker. Get input from your accountant regarding billing cycles, collection letters, timing for sending overdue accounts to a collection agency, and write-offs. **Complete this task before your practice opens so you can train your staff. You want to avoid on-the-spot decision-making about financial policies that should be routine. If you are an existing practice, review your policies regularly.**

33 **Schedule training on billing and collections (FM):** Now that you have tested the claims submission processes for every payer, schedule training on billing and collections for all staff who will be involved. **Although your practice administrator/manager and your billing staff should play lead roles, you, too, should know exactly how your system works. If staff leave your practice or are out of the office unexpectedly, you must know what to do. Complete this task before you open your practice and on an ongoing basis.**

34 **Order patient account statements (FM):** When you order your patient account statements, make sure that the language is clear. If you don't pay attention to details, you may find that your patients confuse statements with bills. **Your practice administrator/manager should handle this task with your input. Complete the task before you open or move your practice.**

35 **Purchase equipment (FM):** You have already made your equipment list and decided what purchases will fit within your budget. **Your practice administrator/manager can place the orders and schedule delivery dates. Complete this task before you open or move your practice.**

36 **Purchase medical supplies (FM):** Your practice administrator/manager can order medical supplies for your office. He/she should investigate purchasing discounts that are available through professional associations and/or directly from vendors. **Complete this task before you open or move your practice.**

37 **Purchase office supplies (FM):** You'll need office supplies as well as medical supplies. Work with your **practice administrator/manager** to make a list. Make sure to investigate opportunities for purchasing discounts. **Complete this task before you open or move your practice.**

38 **Purchase office furniture (FM):** You have already made your list of fixed assets and decided what purchases you can afford. Now you can place your orders. **You or your practice administrator/manager should work with your interior design consultant to order everything so it arrives before the official opening or moving of your practice.**

39 **Activate and test your website (DO):** You have already planned your website. Test its operation to make sure all the functions that you have incorporated into it are working smoothly. **Your practice administrator/manager should handle this task before you open your practice. If you are moving, make sure your website is still working properly.**

40 **Test your e-prescribing capability (DO):** Make sure your e-prescribing capability works smoothly. This function may or may not be part of your practice management or electronic health records system. **Check this capability yourself since it will be an important part of the way you care for patients. Complete the task before you begin seeing patients in your practice.**

41 **Develop a practice brochure, introductory letter, and other materials to announce the opening or new location of your practice (OM):** Your practice brochure says a great deal about you. It communicates your mission, your qualifications, the way in which your office works, and information about your physicians and staff. Keep a hard copy of your brochure in your waiting room and mail it out to announce the opening of your practice. Post the information that is in your brochure on your practice website. **You and your practice administrator/manager should work with a graphic artist and/**

or marketing consultant to complete your brochure before you open or move your practice.

42 **Order business cards, stationery, your practice brochure, and other print material (FM):** You began working on your identity materials early in your planning process, and now you can order business cards, stationery, brochures, and other printed material. **You, your practice administrator/manager, and your graphic artist or marketing consultant can decide what pieces and quantities you need.** Take advantage of quantity discounts, but don't buy as if paper is going out of style. You can always reorder. **Complete this task before you open or move your practice so you can use this material to announce your opening in the community, with medical colleagues, and in your waiting area.**

43 **Order materials for report preparation and filing (FM):** If you prefer paper records to a paperless office, order the specific materials that you need. Your **practice administrator/manager** can order directly from medical practice suppliers. **Complete this task before you open or move your practice so your patient records are organized from the outset.**

44 **Select and engage answering and paging services (DO):** The answering and paging services that you select for your practice should be compatible with any other methods of communication that you have already selected. Ask colleagues in the medical community for the names of reliable services. Then let **your practice administrator/manager obtain relevant details. The answering and paging services should be in place when you open your practice, and you should test them ahead of time to make sure they meet your expectations.**

45 **Draft and finalize an Employee Handbook for your practice (HR):** Your employees are a valuable asset to your practice. You can reduce your exposure to potential legal action if you develop written policies and procedures for hiring, compensation package (wage and salary, benefits), performance evaluation, termination, and conditions of employment. Put this information in an Employee Handbook that you give to all new employees during orientation. **You or your practice administrator/manager should ask an external consultant or your attorney for a sample Employee Handbook before you open your practice. You can later revise the contents to suit your particular situation.** Exhibit A.4 describes the problems that Suburban Plastic Surgery experienced because the practice lacked formal policies and procedures for recruitment and compensation as well as an Employee Handbook.

EXHIBIT A.4 Suburban Plastic Surgery's employee problems

Dr Face had been a successful plastic surgeon at an academic medical center for many years. Eventually he opened his own private practice. His wife, a co-owner, was the interim practice manager. Because Dr Face had spent most of his medical career in an academic medical center where the human resource policies and procedures were already in place, he had little appreciation for the need to create a formal Employee Handbook. He and his wife hired four employees, giving little thought to inconsistencies in the compensation packages. Shortly after the practice opened, Dr and Mrs Face found themselves with mutiny on their hands; the employees were at odds with each other and with the owners because of differences in their working conditions.

51 **Develop a patient information package (DO):** When patients look at your website or come to your office, you want to make sure they understand exactly how your practice works. They need to know what services you provide, how to make appointments, how to get medical advice and test results, and how to renew prescriptions. They need to know your policies regarding confidentiality. They also need to know your financial policies, including payment plans, charging for missed appointments, and collections. **As the owner of your practice, you should determine the policies. Work with your practice administrator/manager to convert them into an information package that is easy to understand. Give patients a hard copy of the package and make it available on your website. Complete this task before you open or move your practice.**

52 **Determine your method(s) for scheduling appointments (DO):** In collaboration with other clinicians in your practice who will take care of patients, decide how you want to schedule appointments. If your website has a function that allows patients to request appointments online, make sure that this feature is working properly. Work with your practice administrator/manager and other staff. **Complete this task before you open or move your practice.**

53 **Decide on your opening date (OM):** By now you should be ready to schedule an official opening or moving date. If you planned properly, your professional credentials are in place, you have hospital privileges, you are part of the managed care and government provider networks that you have chosen, your staff are in place, and your insurance coverage has begun. **Make this decision with your practice administrator/ manager.**

54 **Draft and order cards announcing the opening of your practice (OM):** Now that you have your opening or moving date, you are ready to order announcement cards. **Your practice administrator/manager can assume this responsibility with your input.**

55 **Draft an announcement and place ads in your local newspapers (OM):** Tell your community that you'll soon be open for business, moving to a new location, or offering a new service. Be sure to include your name, address, phone, email address, and welcome to new patients (if you are accepting them). Mention your training and experience and/or participation in managed care plans and government programs. **You decide what your ad says and delegate the details to your practice administrator/ manager. Make sure the ad runs two weeks prior to the date you open or move your practice.**

56 **Develop a list of names to whom you will send the announcement of your opening, move, or offering of a new service (OM):** Begin to build a contact list so you can mail and/or email announcements about your practice and practice newsletters to new and potential patients, referring physicians, healthcare organizations, and the community. The Medical Staff offices of the hospitals where you have privileges can provide lists of other physicians in the community. Chambers of Commerce and other local organizations may also have information. **Your practice administrator/manager can take responsibility for this task, and he/she should do it on an ongoing basis so that your contact list is always current.**

57 **Meet with referring physicians (OM):** As you get closer to your opening, move, or offering of a new service, introduce yourself to other physicians in the community who are potential sources of referral. Depending on your specialty as a primary care physician or specialist, there will be different referral patterns. These patterns will

determine who will be important to you. Make appointments to meet people for coffee or lunch, and offer to go to their places of business. **You are your own best spokesperson, so do this task yourself. Start your networking before you open your practice and continue to do it throughout your medical career.**

58 **Obtain/order periodicals and educational material for your waiting room (OM):** After your patients have made an appointment to seek care from you, the first impression they have of your practice will be your waiting room. Keep the age and sex of your patient population in mind when you order materials. **Your practice administrator/ manager should start this task at least nine weeks before you open or move your practice.** Subscription processing time means you won't receive what you order right away. Exhibit A.5 describes the importance of periodicals in the waiting room of the mammography clinic of a prestigious academic medical center.

EXHIBIT A.5 Mt Shiloh Medical Center's mammography debacle

Mt Shiloh Medical Center was a prestigious academic medical center in the south. It mounted a strong campaign to educate women ages 40 and older about the importance of annual screening mammograms. Sad to say, the mammography waiting room was piled high with magazines on cars, hunting, and fishing. Patients had no access to educational material related to breast cancer. The already anxious atmosphere of the waiting area was unattractive to its patients, and many decided to seek care elsewhere in the community.

59 **Obtain/amend membership in state and county medical societies and in professional associations (OM):** Throughout your medical career, you'll want to make sure you are not practicing in isolation from your medical colleagues. Your county and state medical societies and professional associations of physicians in your specialty can help you remain up-to-date on important issues and develop connections both within your community and throughout the state. Particularly if you are a solo practice or a small provider, these organizations often offer education and assistance in practice management as well as information on important healthcare political issues. **Make these contacts yourself. If you do this task before you set your practice up, you may get some good suggestions.**

60 **Train your employees on your practice management system, web-based communication, EHR, and e-prescribing systems (HR):** As you approach the opening or move of your practice, train your staff on the systems available from different vendors. Consider cross-training people so they can cover for each other when someone is out sick or on vacation. Ask the vendors to do the training at your practice site, and after you open, take advantage of the free or fee-based follow-up user group training available at the vendor site. **You and your practice administrator/manager already scheduled this staff training with your vendors. Be sure to complete the training before you open or move your practice. You'll have employee turnover and your vendors will upgrade their systems, so repeat this training regularly.**

61 **Train your employees on your billing system (FM):** There are many available options for billing and collections. If you purchase one of the newer and more comprehensive practice management systems, the billing and collections functions may reduce the workload for your staff. If you decide to outsource billing and collections, your staff may be responsible for some but not all of billing and collections. Or, you may be

doing both billing and collection in your office. Whatever your decision for your practice, make sure that all of your physicians and employees are clear on procedures for coding, billing, and collections. **Although both your practice administrator/ manager and billing staff will play a big role in your billing and collections, you're the practice owner, and ultimately you need to know exactly what is going on. Complete this training before you open or move your practice. Repeat the training regularly so new employees know exactly what to do.**

62 **Train your employees on HIPAA compliance (C):** HIPAA compliance is a part of doing business. You must designate HIPAA Privacy and HIPAA Security Officials; these can be the same person or different individuals. Train all members of your workforce, including physicians and employees, on the basics of the HIPAA Privacy and Security Rules. **Ask an external consultant and your practice administrator/manager to conduct the HIPAA training before you open your practice. Make sure you incorporate HIPAA training into orientation for new employees and do a refresher at least annually. Complete the initial training before you open your practice and do annual updates.**

63 **Obtain any manuals that you will need for your office (DO):** Although more and more information is available on line, you should still have basic manuals available in your office. For example, maintain written documentation for Medicare, Medicaid, coding, and on each managed care plan with which you contract. Your practice administrator/manager should regularly search key websites for new information that you can then download and make available for your staff. **Your practice manager should begin this task before you open your practice. He/she should continue to make sure that your written manuals are up-to-date.**

64 **Set up accounting systems for accounts payable, petty cash, and bank reconciliations (FM):** Your accountant can help you set up the accounting systems that you need to run your practice. As the practice owner, make sure that you are involved in this process. Your practice administrator/manager should assume a lead role. **Complete this task before you open or relocate your practice.**

65 **Train your employees on your accounting systems (FM):** Make sure that your practice administrator/manager trains your employees on your accounts payable, petty cash, and bank reconciliation systems. **He/she should complete this task before you open your practice. Provide refresher training on a regular basis.**

66 **Prepare employee personnel files (HR/C):** Make sure you set up employee personnel files and keep them in a secure place. You are required to comply with HIPAA not only as a medical practice, but also as employer, so you don't want your employee files accessible to anyone other than your practice administrator/manager and one of the physician owners. **Your practice administrator/manager should complete this task before your practice opens.**

67 **Train your employees on operating policies and procedures (DO):** Make sure that your operating policies and procedures are clear to all your employees. Clarify your entire work flow process before you open your doors or move. If you are currently in practice, regularly review the operating policies and procedures to make sure they are effective and that your staff understands them. **Your practice administrator/manager should take responsibility for the training, and he/she should do it before you open or move, and then on a regular basis.**

68 **Begin developing a Quality/Quality Improvement plan (DO):** All physicians think

they provide excellent care, but in the future, that confidence won't be sufficient. Professional credentialing organizations and public and private payers will require proof of the care you are providing to individual patients and for groups of patients. You will also be expected to benchmark your practice against others and against evidence-based standards. You or another physician in your practice should learn about quality and quality improvement and develop a plan for your practice. Ultimately, everyone needs to buy into the plan, but somebody needs to start the ball rolling. **Begin your work on quality and quality improvement before you start your practice or move to a new location, and continue it throughout your career.**

69 **Plan the details of your opening (PO):** Plan a nice celebration for the opening or move of your practice. Send out invitations and information on your practice to the medical community, to representatives of hospitals where you have privileges, and to others in the community who are potential sources of business for you. Make sure you have available information on your practice and business cards. **Work with your practice manager to make your plans.**

70 **Opening or moving day!**

List of Additional Appendices Appearing only on the Website

The following Appendices appear on the website www.radcliffeoxford.com/medicalpractice mangement

Appendix B: Business Planning Questions
Appendix C: Sample Surveys
Appendix D: Financial Management Resources
Appendix E: Revenue Cycle Management Aids
Appendix F: Sample Performance Evaluation Program
Appendix G: Sample Consulting Proposals and Agreements
Appendix H: Quality of Care Digest
Appendix I: Resources to Use When Acquiring Information Technology
Appendix J: A Glossary of HIPAA Terms
Appendix K: Additional HIPAA Compliance Resources

Index

accountability
  decisions 11–16
  HIPAA 136–7
accountants, role 43, 46, 47
accounting 42–4
  accrual accounting 44
  balance sheets 43, 44
  cash flow statements 43
  income statements 42–3
  lag 43–4
  outsourcing 105–8
accrual accounting 44
action steps, business planning 22
activities categories 1–3
affiliation decisions 9–10
aged trial balance, revenue cycle
  management 57
agencies
  collection agencies 67, 105–8
  recruitment 90
agreements
  consultants 116
  information technology 142–3
Anti-Kickback Act 152–3
appendices
  additional 185
  steps for creating a strong
   foundation 171–84
application service provider (ASP),
  information technology 135
applications, information technology
  130–1
ASP see application service provider
assumptions
  budgets/budgeting 40
  business planning 20–1

background checks, recruitment
  76
bad debt
  budgets/budgeting 42
  revenue cycle management 57–8
balance sheets, accounting 43, 44
Beakman Ear, Nose, and Throat,
  revenue cycle management 56
benchmarks, revenue cycle
  management 56–9

benefits package, human resources
  (HR) 78–9
billing/collections
  checklist 107–8
  outsourcing 105–8
bonding, Financial Management
  (FM) 46
BPO see business processing
  outsourcing
Bridges to Excellence (BTE), quality
  of care 122
Brown Street Family Medicine,
  information technology 109
BTE see Bridges to Excellence
budgets/budgeting 39–42
  assumptions 40
  bad debt 42
  business planning 21–2
  capital budget 22
  contractual allowance 42
  discounting 42
  fees 41–2
  operating budget 21–2
  steps 39–42
  volume projections 40–1
business, decisions 14–15
business planning 17–26
  action steps 22
  assumptions 20–1
  budgets/budgeting 21–2
  challenges 26
  contents of plan 18–22
  expenses 21–2
  financial planning 18, 111–12
  goal categories 18
  implementation plan 18, 22
  information gathering 24
  keys to successful 25–6
  leadership 24
  marketing 29
  mission 18
  participants 23–4
  reasons 17–18
  revenue projections 21–2
  steps 22, 24–5
  strategic plan 18–21
  successful 25–6

  timing 24
  using 23
  values 18
  vision 18
  volume projections 21–2
  worksheet 19–20
business processing outsourcing
  (BPO), human resources (HR)
  110–11

C see Compliance
capital budget, budgets/budgeting
  22
Capitol Internal Medicine,
  reimbursement problems 172
cash flow statements, accounting 43
cash management 45–6
centers of excellence, quality of care
  120–1
CEUs see continuing education
  units
challenges
  business planning 26
  Cornwallis Internal Medicine
   11
  information technology 131–3
charges see fees
checklist
  billing/collections 107–8
  discharges 83–4
  disciplinary action 83–4
  information technology 109
  managed care consultants 105
  orientation, employee 77
  physician issues 89–99
Civil Monetary Penalties Act 150
client-site server, information
  technology 135
clinical operations, decisions 14–15
clinical outcomes see Improving
  Healthcare Delivery and Clinical
  Outcomes
colleagues, marketing 33–4
collection agencies, revenue cycle
  management 67, 105–8
collection/billings, outsourcing
  105–8

compensation package
  human resources (HR) 78–9,
    94–6
  physician issues 94–6
competition, marketing 28
Compliance (C)
  see also corporate compliance
    areas 156
  HIPAA 136–7, 159–69
  regulations 3
constraints, marketing 37–8
consultants 113–16
  agreements 116
  characteristics 114–15
  charges 116
  finding 115
  hiring 113–16
  managing 113–16
  perspective 114
  Tall Oaks ObGyn 114
continuing education units
  (CEUs), human resources (HR)
  78
contractual allowance, budgets/
  budgeting 42
controls, Financial Management
  (FM) 45–6, 47–8, 49–51
Cornwallis Internal Medicine,
  challenges 11
corporate compliance 147–57
  see also Compliance (C)
  advantages 148
  Anti-Kickback Act 152–3
  Civil Monetary Penalties Act
    150
  defining 147
  FCA 150
  laws 150–4
  legal issues 150–4
  maintaining 154–6
  penalties for non-compliance
    150–4
  planning 147–8, 154–6
  programs 154–6
  regulations 150–4
  risk areas 149
  safe harbors 153–4
  Stark Self-Referral Prohibitions
    150–3
  steps 154–6
Corporation, legal entity 8
criminal checks, recruitment 76

decision-making, influencers' role,
  healthcare 28
decisions
  accountability 11–16
  affiliation 9–10
  business 14–15
  clinical operations 14–15

financial management (FM)
  12–13
  governance 14
  human resource management 13
  information technology 14
  marketing 13–14
  organizational dynamics 14
  planning 13–14
  practice structure 11–16
  professional responsibility
    15–16
  relationships 10–11
  responsibilities 15–16
  risk management 14
demographics
  human resources (HR) 85–7
  marketing 34
departures
  checklist 99
  human resources (HR) 83–5,
    98–9
  physician issues 98–9
diabetic patients, marketing 34
discharges
  checklist 83–4
  human resources (HR) 83–5
disciplinary action
  checklist 83–4
  human resources (HR) 82–4
discounting, budgets/budgeting 42
discrimination, job 70–1
disease management, quality of care
  120
dissolution, legal issues 172
diversity, human resources (HR)
  85–7
DO *see* Improving Healthcare
  Delivery and Clinical Outcomes
documenting
  HIPAA 167
  quality of care 126

e-prescribing, information
  technology 131
Eagle Surgical Associates, physician
  issues 171
EBM *see* evidence-based medicine
effectiveness, measuring
  marketing 30, 36
  quality of care 122–3
EHR *see* electronic health records
electronic health records (EHR)
  information technology 130–1,
    133–6
  marketing 32
  quality of care 119
  revenue cycle management 66
Empire Medical Associates, billing/
  collections 107
employers, marketing 35

employment *see* human resources
  (HR)
enhancing revenue, revenue cycle
  management 66
environment, workplace 80
ethical constraints, marketing 37–8
evaluation
  information technology 143–4
  performance, employee 82, 96–8
  physician issues 96–8
evidence-based medicine (EBM),
  quality of care 121
expenses, business planning 21–2
external help
  HIPAA 168
  revenue cycle management 64
external marketing 33–5

facilities, workplace 80
False Claims Act (FCA) 150
fees
  see also revenue cycle
    management; revenue
    projections
  budgets/budgeting 41–2
Financial Management (FM) 2,
  39–51
  accountants 43, 46, 47
  accounting 42–4
  advice, seeking 49–51
  bonding 46
  budgets/budgeting 39–42
  cash management 45–6
  concerns 47–8
  controls 45–6, 47–8, 49–51
  decisions 12–13
  fraud protection 46
  information review 47, 48–9
  internal controls 45–6, 47–8,
    49–51
  leadership 47–8
  learning 48
  overhead expenses 44–5
  planning 46
  practice management
    (operations and clinical) 44
  problems 47–8, 49–51
  reporting systems 47–8
  responsibilities 45–51
  reviewing information 47, 48–9
  Stonebrook Internal Medicine
    50–1
financial planning
  see also budgets/budgeting
  business planning 18
  outsourcing 111–12
  suggestions 111–12
Florence Family Medicine,
  information technology 145
FM *see* Financial Management

foundation, practice 1–3
foundation, steps for creating a
    strong 171–84
fraud protection, Financial
    Management (FM) 46

General Partnership, legal entity 7
generational issues, human resources
    (HR) 85–7
goal categories, business planning 18
goals
    information technology 137
    recruitment 72–3
Gornish Medical Group, HIPAA
    163, 164
governance, decisions 14
governments, local, marketing 35
grievances, human resources (HR)
    81
Group Practices without Walls,
    affiliation decisions 9

Happy Pediatrics
    dissolution 172
    information technology 134
    legal issues 172
Health Insurance Portability and
    Accountability Act (HIPAA)
    basic information 165
    benefits 160
    breadth of coverage 162
    commitment 167
    comparisons 162–3
    compliance 159–69
    concepts 169
    degree of direction 162
    documenting 167
    enforcement 161
    external help 168
    gap analysis 166
    Gornish Medical Group 163,
        164
    help sources 168
    history 160
    information technology 136–7
    management 167
    management discretion 163
    marketing 37
    monitoring 167
    officials 164–5
    overview 159–69
    personnel 164–5
    policies/procedures 166
    purpose 160
    responsibilities 163
    steps 165–7
    successful compliance factors
        167–8
    Tall Oaks Internal Medicine 165
    timetable 160–1

training 166–7
    workforce involvement 168
health plans
    see also managed care companies
    marketing 35
healthcare delivery see Improving
    Healthcare Delivery and Clinical
    Outcomes
help sources
    HIPAA 168
    revenue cycle management 64,
        68
HIPAA see Health Insurance
    Portability and Accountability Act
hospitals
    local 34
    marketing 34
human resources (HR) 69–88
    see also recruitment
    benefits package 78–9
    BPO 110–11
    CEUs 78
    compensation package 78–9,
        94–6
    decisions 13
    demographics 85–7
    departures 83–5, 98–9
    discharges 84–5
    disciplinary action 82–4
    discrimination 70–1
    diversity 85–7
    environment, workplace 80
    facilities 80
    generational issues 85–7
    grievances 81
    information technology 86, 90
    job descriptions 74
    job offer 76–7
    job requirements 73–4
    job stability 81
    legal issues 69–72
    orientation, employee 77–8, 93
    outsourcing 110–11
    PEO 110–11
    performance evaluation 82,
        96–8
    problems 110, 180
    recruitment 72–7
    resignations 84–5
    resources 87–8, 100–1
    sexual harassment 71–2
    Suburban Plastic Surgery 180
    total compensation package
        78–9
    training 78
    wages/salaries 78–9, 94–6

implementation plan
    business planning 18, 22
    information technology 143

importance issues, practice settings
    5–6
Improving Healthcare Delivery and
    Clinical Outcomes (DO) 2–3
income statements, accounting 42–3
Independent Practice Associations
    (IPAs), affiliation decisions 9
indicators, revenue cycle
    management 56–9
information gathering, business
    planning 24
information review, Financial
    Management (FM) 47, 48–9
information technology 129–46
    agreements 142–3
    applications 130–1
    ASP 135
    Brown Street Family Medicine
        109
    challenges 131–3
    checklist 109
    client-site server 135
    decisions 14
    e-prescribing 131
    EHR 130–1, 133–6
    evaluation 143–4
    evolution 135
    Florence Family Medicine 145
    goals 137
    Happy Pediatrics 134
    HIPAA 136–7
    human resources (HR) 86, 90
    impact 129
    implementation plan 143
    implementing 131–3
    inventory 133
    learning from experiences 144–5
    outsourcing 108–9
    planning 131–3, 143
    PMS 130–1, 133–6
    practice profile 138
    priorities 137
    quality of care 119
    questions 133–6
    red flags 141
    Red River Urology Associates
        133–4
    references 142
    resources 138–9, 145
    responsibilities 134
    revenue cycle management 67–8
    RFI 139
    RFP 139
    site visits 142
    steps 136–44
    successful 144
    task force 137–8
    timing 133–4
    Vendor Q 136
    vendors, comparing 140–2

information technology (*continued*)
  vendors, identifying 138–9
  vendors, selecting 142–3
  websites 36, 131
  White Ice Internal Medicine 132
Institute of Medicine (IOM), quality
  of care recommendations 118–20
Integrated Delivery Systems,
  affiliation decisions 10
internal controls, Financial
  Management (FM) 45–6
internal marketing 32–3
interviews, recruitment 75–6
inventory, information technology
  133
IOM *see* Institute of Medicine
IPAs *see* Independent Practice
  Associations

job descriptions, recruitment 74
job offer, recruitment 76–7
job requirements, recruitment 73–4
job stability, human resources (HR)
  81

lag, accounting 43–4
leadership
  business planning 24
  Financial Management (FM)
    47–8
Leapfrog Group, quality of care
  121–2
legal constraints
  marketing 37–8
  *Medical Group Practice, Legal
    and Administrative Guide*
    37–8
legal decisions 6–9
legal entities 7–9
legal issues
  Anti-Kickback Act 152–3
  Civil Monetary Penalties Act
    150
  corporate compliance 150–4
  dissolution 172
  FCA 150
  Happy Pediatrics 172
  HIPAA 136–7, 159–69
  human resources (HR) 69–72
  physician issues 89–92, 171
  practice dissolution 172
  recruitment 89–92, 171
  Stark Self-Referral Prohibitions
    150–3
Limited Liability Company, legal
  entity 8
Limited Liability Partnership, legal
  entity 8
Limited Partnership, legal entity 8
local governments, marketing 35

mammography
  marketing 182
  Mt Shiloh Medical Center 182
managed care
  checklist 105
  outsourcing 103–5
managed care companies
  reimbursement, maximizing
    60–4, 172
  reimbursement problems 172
  revenue cycle management 60–4
managed care consultants, checklist
  105
management
  MGMA 60
  practice management
    (operations and clinical) 44
management, organization and *see*
  Organization and Management
Management Service Organizations
  (MSOs), affiliation decisions 9
Managing Staff and Outside
  Resources (HR) 3
  see also human resources (HR)
marketing 27–38
  attainability 30
  attributes 29–33
  business planning 29
  colleagues 33–4
  competition 28
  constraints 37–8
  current patients 32
  decisions 13–14
  defining 27
  demographic groups 34
  diabetic patients 34
  effectiveness 30, 36
  EHR 32
  employers 35
  ethical constraints 37–8
  expertise, external 36
  external 33–5
  governments, local 35
  health plans 35
  HIPAA 37
  hospitals, local 34
  internal 32–3
  legal constraints 37–8
  mammography 182
  measuring effectiveness 30, 36
  media contacts 34
  *Medical Group Practice, Legal
    and Administrative Guide* 37–8
  Mt Shiloh Medical Center 182
  patients, current 32
  patients, potential 33
  patients' viewpoint 28–9
  PHI 37
  programs 29–33
  public agencies 35

reasons 27
recruitment 75
Red Cross Red Shield of
  Georgia 35
rewarding 30–1
schools 35
simplicity 29–30
specificity 29–30
Student Success Center (SSC)
  31
target groups 31–2, 34
timing 31
websites 36, 131
workforce 30, 32–3
maximizing patient revenue,
  revenue cycle management 60,
  64–6
maximizing reimbursement
  managed care companies 60–4
  revenue cycle management 60–6
measuring effectiveness
  marketing 30, 36
  quality of care 122–3
media contacts, marketing 34
Medical Group Management
  Association (MGMA) 12
  recruitment 75
  revenue cycle management 60
*Medical Group Practice, Legal and
  Administrative Guide*, marketing
  37–8
Medicare, revenue cycle
  management 62–3
MGMA *see* Medical Group
  Management Association
mission
  business planning 18
  recruitment 72–3
MSOs *see* Management Service
  Organizations
Mt. Shiloh Medical Center,
  marketing 182
Multi-specialty Group, practice
  type 6

National Committee for Quality
  Assurance (NCQA), quality of
  care 121
national standards, revenue cycle
  management 62–3
NCQA *see* National Committee for
  Quality Assurance
NDRO *see* net days receivable
  outstanding
negotiations, revenue cycle
  management 63–4
net charges to cash collections,
  revenue cycle management 57
net collection rate, revenue cycle
  management 57

net days receivable outstanding (NDRO), revenue cycle management 57
Networks, affiliation decisions 10

office-based settings, quality of care 122
Organization and Management (OM) 1–2, 5–16
organizational dynamics, decisions 14
orientation, employee
    checklist 77
    human resources (HR) 77–8, 93
    physician issues 93
outsourcing 103–12
    accounting 105–8
    billing/collections 67, 105–8
    financial planning 111–12
    human resources (HR) 110–11
    information technology 108–9
    managed care 103–5
    revenue cycle management 67, 105–8
overhead expenses, Financial Management (FM) 44–5

P4P see Pay-for-Performance
PA see Professional Association
patient revenue, maximizing 60, 64–6
patients
    current 32
    judging practices 28–9
    marketing 28–9, 32, 33
    potential 33
Pay-for-Performance (P4P), quality of care 122
payer-specific information, revenue cycle management 58–9
PC see Professional Corporation
penalties, non-compliance 150–4
PEO see professional employer organization
performance evaluation
    human resources (HR) 82, 96–8
    physician issues 96–8
personal interviews, recruitment 75–6
PHI see protected health information
Physician Hospital Organizations (PHOs), affiliation decisions 9
physician issues 89–101
    checklist 89–99
    compensation package 94–6
    concerns 91–2
    departures 98–9
    Eagle Surgical Associates 171
    evaluation 96–8

legal issues 89–92, 171
orientation, employee 93
performance evaluation 96–8
questions 91
recruitment 89–92, 171
resources 100–1
retention 92–3
planning
    see also business planning
    corporate compliance 147–8, 154–6
    decisions 13–14
    Financial Management (FM) 46
    financial planning 18, 111–12
    information technology 131–3, 143
PMS see practice management system
practice dissolution, legal issues 172
practice guidelines, quality of care 121
practice management system (PMS), information technology 130–1, 133–6
practice profile, information technology 138
practice settings, importance issues 5–6
practice structure, decisions 11–16
practice types 5–6
prescribing, e-prescribing 131
priorities
    information technology 137
    recruitment 72–3
Privacy Rules/Security Rules, HIPAA 136–7, 159–69
Professional Association (PA), legal entity 8–9
Professional Corporation (PC), legal entity 8–9
professional employer organization (PEO), human resources (HR) 110–11
professional responsibility, decisions 15–16
protected health information (PHI), marketing 37
protecting revenue, revenue cycle management 66
public agencies, marketing 35

quality of care 117–27
    BTE 122
    centers of excellence 120–1
    defining 118
    disease management 120
    documenting 126
    EBM 121
    EHR 119

    examples 120–2
    information technology 119
    initiatives 123
    IOM recommendations 118–20
    Leapfrog Group 121–2
    learning 123–4
    measuring effectiveness 122–3
    NCQA 121
    objectivity 125–6
    office-based settings 122
    organizing 126
    outcomes 125–6
    P4P 122
    practice guidelines 121
    programs 120–2
    public/private initiatives 123
    responsibilities 124
    suggestions 123–6

recruitment 72–7
    see also human resources (HR)
    agencies 90
    background checks 76
    criminal checks 76
    goals 72–3
    interviews 75–6
    job descriptions 74
    job offer 76–7
    job requirements 73–4
    legal issues 89–92, 171
    marketing 75
    MGMA 75
    mission 72–3
    physician issues 89–92, 171
    priorities 72–3
    recruitment firms 90
    references 76
    resumés 75
    retention 92–3
    Swan River Ear, Nose, & Throat 89–90
    values 72–3
Red Cross Red Shield of Georgia, marketing 35
red flags, IT vendors 141
Red River Urology Associates, information technology 133–4
references
    information technology 142
    recruitment 76
regulations
    see also legal issues
    Compliance (C) 3
    corporate compliance 150–4
reimbursement, maximizing, managed care companies 60–4, 172
reimbursement problems
    Capitol Internal Medicine 172
    managed care companies 172

relationships, colleagues, decisions 10–11
relationships, working, revenue cycle management 61
reporting systems, Financial Management (FM) 47–8
Request for Information (RFI), information technology 139
Request for Proposal (RFP), information technology 139
resignations, human resources (HR) 84–5
resources
    human resources (HR) 87–8, 100–1
    information technology 138–9, 145
    physician issues 100–1
responsibilities
    decisions 15–16
    Financial Management (FM) 45–51
    HIPAA 163
    information technology 134
    quality of care 124
    revenue cycle management 55–6
resumés, recruitment 75
retention
    physician issues 92–3
    recruitment 92–3
revenue cycle management 53–68
    see also fees
    Beakman Ear, Nose, and Throat 56
    benchmarks 56–9
    billing/collections 105–8
    collection agencies 67, 105–8
    EHR 66
    Empire Medical Associates 107
    enhancing revenue 66
    external help 64
    help sources 64, 68
    indicators 56–9
    information technology 67–8
    managed care companies 60–4
    maximizing patient revenue 60, 64–6
    maximizing reimbursement 60–6
    Medicare 62–3
    MGMA 60
    national standards 62–3
    negotiations 63–4
    outsourcing 105–8
    patient revenue 60, 64–6
    protecting revenue 66

relationships 61
responsibilities 55–6
Short Hills Pulmonary Consultants 54
St Nicholas Health Plan 61
standards, national 62–3
steps 53–5
revenue projections
    see also fees
    business planning 21–2
reviewing information, Financial Management (FM) 47, 48–9
RFI see Request for Information
RFP see Request for Proposal
risk areas
    see also corporate compliance
    physician practices 149
risk management, decisions 14

safe harbors, corporate compliance 153–4
salaries/wages
    human resources (HR) 78–9, 94–6
    physician issues 94–6
schools, marketing 35
Security Rules/Privacy Rules, HIPAA 136–7, 159–69
sexual harassment, workplace 71–2
Short Hills Pulmonary Consultants, revenue cycle management 54
Single Specialty Group, practice type 6
site visits, information technology 142
Sole Proprietorship, legal entity 7
Solo practice, practice type 6
SSC see Student Success Center
St Nicholas Health Plan, revenue cycle management 61
staff management see Managing Staff and Outside Resources
standards, national, revenue cycle management 62–3
Stark Self-Referral Prohibitions 150–3
steps
    budgets/budgeting 39–42
    business planning 22, 24–5
    corporate compliance 154–6
    HIPAA 165–7
    information technology 136–44
    revenue cycle management 53–5
    strong foundation 171–84
Stonebrook Internal Medicine, Financial Management (FM) 50–1

strategic plan, business planning 18–21
strong foundation, steps 171–84
Student Success Center (SSC), marketing 31
Suburban Plastic Surgery, human resources (HR) 180
support, workforce 30
Swan River Ear, Nose, & Throat, recruitment 89–90

Tall Oaks Internal Medicine, HIPAA 165
Tall Oaks ObGyn, consultants 114
target groups, marketing 31–2, 34
task force, information technology 137–8
telephone interviews, recruitment 75
timing
    business planning 24
    information technology 133–4
    marketing 31
total compensation package, human resources (HR) 78–9
training
    HIPAA 166–7
    human resources (HR) 78
types of practice 5–6

values
    business planning 18
    recruitment 72–3
Vendor Q, information technology 136
vision, business planning 18
volume projections
    budgets/budgeting 40–1
    business planning 21–2

wages/salaries
    human resources (HR) 78–9, 94–6
    physician issues 94–6
websites, marketing 36, 131
White Ice Internal Medicine, information technology 132
workforce
    marketing 30, 32–3
    support 30
workforce involvement, HIPAA 168
workplace
    environment 80
    facilities 80
    sexual harassment 71–2
worksheet, business planning 19–20